Contents

Contents

Figures and Tables

Preface

This book is concerned with the identification of problems that currently beset the relationship between doctors and their patients. It examines the roles that science, ethics and the humanities may be playing in the genesis and the correction of poor communication. The essence of medical practice and the justification for medical research still reside in the individual relationship between a doctor and a patient. The current fashion for managerialism in medicine may help to resolve some of the important issues that exist in the public domain, but it will do nothing to resolve the conflicts that arise in the interpersonal domain. The perspective is that of the clinician, rather than that of the patient. The patient's view has been well stated by Kay Toombs,[1] a philosopher who suffers from multiple sclerosis. I do not pretend to have found the answers, but I think that I have at least defined some of the important issues.

The book begins by reviewing the signs of discontent within and around the medical profession, and the imperfection of the data which clinicians use when they make decisions. The first chapter makes the point that modern Western medicine needs to measure what it is doing to quality of life, rather than quantity of life. Chapter 2 examines the complexity of the clinical process, using models that were first proposed by Sir Karl Popper. As the discussion develops, it becomes clear that some of medicine's current communication problems are actually caused by the science which has been at the heart of medical progress in the last 150 years. The scientific process within medicine is analysed in some detail. This leads to a discussion of the interdependence of science and clinical practice and the importance of medical research. While this orientation toward science is seen as important and ultimately constructive, there are hidden problems. One of these problems is the double-edged impact of authority in medicine. Research directors and senior doctors have an aura of respect and power. There are dangers in accepting beliefs because they are handed down by accepted authorities within the collegial structure of medicine. It is easy to accept that a course of action or an explanation is the 'best' because an eminent figure has endorsed it. The fact remains that courses of action in the biological sciences, particularly medicine, have probable rather than determinate outcomes. The concept of probability in medicine is therefore discussed in some detail, in chapter 5, which emphasises that the difficulty of communicating uncertainty is the basis of at least part of the failure of the doctor–patient relationship.

Would better data solve these problems, as some writers claim? How would we combine information about the probability of success or failure of a treatment with outcomes that reflect the impact of the treatment on quality of life and autonomy, together with the costs of treatment? This question is examined in some detail in chapter 6. It is clear that excellent data will help communication, but still cannot guarantee its quality.

If accurate numbers cannot provide the answer, can doctors look to ethics to help them in their relations with patients, since ethics are supposed to regulate the way that doctors deal properly with their patients? The ethical movement has been important in medicine, particularly since the Second World War, and has become one of the essential components of any profession (discussed in chapter 7). Bioethics has also emerged as a 'specialty' in the last 10 to 20 years. The ethical movement has, like the scientific movement, contributed significantly to the way that late 20th century medicine is practised and the way that it conducts its research. But ethical standards cannot be enforced. Once they become legislative requirements, they move from the ethical domain to the legal. This is particularly true of the issue of informed consent, which is examined separately, in chapter 9. Like good data, ethical discussion can help, but it cannot ensure good communication. Bringing science and ethics together, however, can perhaps achieve more than each alone, by providing narrower ranges of probability and a framework for discussion along lines recommended by the profession itself.

Even the approach that combines science and ethics leaves something out. The art of communicating with patients presupposes a level of language skills and of human understanding which medical faculties emphasise, but seldom teach. Hermeneutics is the study of interpretation. The term was originally used to describe the study and interpretation of Biblical texts, but now has a wide connotation which covers secular interpretation, communication and meaning. It is derived from the name of Hermes, in Greek mythology patron of the arts and eloquence. (He was also patron of herdsmen and thieves, but 'hermeneutic' refers only to his more respectable patronage.) Modern hermeneutic philosophers have examined the complex processes that occur as people talk and change their conversation to text — a process which is closely followed by doctors taking medical histories. An understanding of these complexities may help doctors and patients to communicate more comfortably with one another. This is the subject of chapter 10.

Finally, in chapter 11 the book enters a plea for an increased emphasis on the humanities within medicine. It is unlikely that students can be taught by a medical faculty to enjoy and assimilate the arts, but the selection processes for entering medicine can be adjusted so that language skills and talents in the humanities are given as much weight as scientific and mathematical achievement. There is evidence that this weighting will do no harm, and that language skills predict 'success' in medicine at least as well as skills in the sciences. It is suggested that medical teaching would best be served by using a problem-oriented system in the clinical years. Each learning episode would involve using the relevant science to handle the ethical and hermeneutic issues.

This book may be best understood by medical graduates of some seniority and by more general readers with an interest in education, sociology, health policy and the philosophy and anthropology of medicine. Lawyers and politicians may appreciate the book's messages, attitudes and insights when they formulate legislation and health policies. I hope that medical teachers will find the messages important enough to want to teach them to their students. I would not favour teaching these values in a medical course by a rigid pedagogic program, but a program which is so much interleaved with the rest of clinical teaching as to be inseparable from it. Each teaching or learning episode should include some acknowledgment of relevant ethical, epistemological and ontological issues, so that medical graduates accept the uncertain grounds of their 'knowledge', and learn to live as comfortably as possible with making decisions and offering advice against the background of a certain degree of doubt. An example of a teaching package of this kind is appended to the book. It may mean little to those without medical training, but it is designed to illustrate how the value-laden aspects of medical education can be interwoven with the necessary science, without strain.

A glossary at the end of the book contains explanations of the technical terms and subjects discussed in the book. In most cases, a term or concept is explained the first time it is mentioned in the text. The glossary provides readers with an easily-accessible explanation for future reference.

I am more grateful than I can really say to those who read and criticised as they were written the papers on which this book is based, and who kindly encouraged me to publish some of them in a variety of journals. I am particularly grateful to Professors Stephen Leeder, Cres Eastman, Peter Castaldi, John Stewart and Les Bokey, and to Drs Jeremy Chapman and Noel Tait for their patience and their refusal to dismiss me as misguided, and to Dr Kim Paul for her anthropological insights. In the United States, Dr Martin Adson and Dr Pat Adson were consistently supportive and constructively critical. My wife Penelope — who knows from experience that the medical profession has problems with its communication skills — was patient, helpful, tolerant, and optimistic. I am also grateful to the editors of the *Mayo Clinic Proceedings* and *Theoretical Surgery* for permission to use the text of articles published in those journals. In particular, material from chapter 9 is in publication in the journal *Theoretical Surgery*. Professor Wilfrid Lorenz of Marburg, in particular, was immensely helpful, both as an editor and a mentor. His devotion to the new science of decision theory is well-known, and no one has done more to proclaim the value of combining science with philosophy in this field.

Finally, I thank Phillipa McGuinness and the rest of the staff of Cambridge University Press in Sydney, Australia, from the bottom of my heart for their persistence and their gentleness in their handling of a crabby old professor of surgery with ideas above his station. I have enjoyed our collaboration, and I have learned a great deal about writing on matters that are neither purely medical nor strictly scientific.

NOTES

1. Toombs SK. The meaning of illness. A phenomenological account of the different perspectives of physician and patient. Dordrecht: Kluwer Academic Publishers, 1992.

1

Confronting the Present: Confronting the Future

Medicine presumably began because of the human perception of individual human suffering, and the slow realisation that humans could influence the functions of the body. The first healers may have been wise men and women who were thought of as magicians because of their ability to interpret and manipulate. The abilities to interpret and manipulate are as important now as they were thousands of years ago, when they were first used to prolong life or improve the quality of life. The mission of medicine has not changed, but its methods have. The connection between modern medicine and its still-valid roots is found in the language that connects doctor and patient — language that should be precise, economical, considered and flexible.

But there is something very wrong with present medicine and medical practice. Over three decades after graduating, I have to say that things have changed — and this is not solely a reflection of advancing age and increasing conservatism. Much of the change has been for the better. Conditions that would have taken life or reduced its quality can be treated or palliated far more effectively than they could when I graduated. The leukaemias and lymphatic cancers were then effectively sentences of death within a relatively short time, and are now potentially curable. Major trauma carried a dreadful mortality. In the 1950s

62% of patients with liver injuries died. Now, only 20% will die, and most of those from associated brain injury. Surgeons can transplant kidneys, liver, heart and lungs, pancreas and small bowel. Plastic surgeons transpose skin, bone and muscle from one part of the body to another in order to restore tissue damaged by injuries or burns, or to fill the deformities created by other surgeons removing large cancers. Medical scientists are involved in a massive project to map the human genome, and gene therapy is already available for a few disorders. The life expectancy at birth in Western countries has increased by about 26 years since the start of the century.

And yet it seems that no one is really happy with the way that medicine is practised, nor with the way the profession has concentrated on the immensely productive science that underpins the advances in modern medicine. Hafferty and Salloway[1] wrote 'The profession of medicine has changed dramatically in 75 years. Despite the commitment of individual practitioners to the highest ideals of professionalism, the profession itself has lost privilege, power, and public reputation.' Science has shaped the image of the profession in the late 20th century, and there is a sense in which that science seems to be blamed for failings that are certainly perceived and are sometimes articulated in lawsuits, newspaper articles and television programs. Further, the science of medicine generates the technology of medicine with all its enormous costs — costs which probably do more to raise the national expenditure on health than any other component. It does not seem to matter how much a nation spends on health. The amount is always too much, and government wants to control and to reduce it, while insisting that full services are maintained.

The public perceives medicine to be too impersonal. Government sees it as too expensive. The profession, more particularly its university faculties, perceives problems that are hard to define precisely. These misgivings concern the content of what is taught, the imbalance between teaching and learning and the lack of real concern among the faculty for the values that should provide the moral and intellectual bases of medical research and practice. There is so much information bombarding professionals that it is no longer possible for specialists to remain completely up to date within their area of specialism, and yet little is taught about information technology or the methods of critical appraisal of evidence. University teachers and their clinical colleagues identify poor communication skills in graduates as one of the greatest failings of the medical curriculum, and medical consumer groups would generally agree with that judgment. Traditional general practice until the Second World War had a much better public image because of the hermeneutic skills of practitioners. There were not so many effective treatments then as there are now, but few people now feel so warmly toward the medical profession. Judged by modern standards, the practitioners of those days were far more paternalistic, and much less regardful of the need for informed consent. They knew what was good for their patients, and how much it was good to tell them. (Even in the mid 1960s, my 32-year-old sister was not told that she had metastatic bowel cancer until just before she died.) Auditing and peer review were unknown. The publication lists of eminent physicians and surgeons were usually very brief. In short, they knew less, they were able to do less in the way of treatment, they had few diagnostic tests of real value, and their ethical code emphasised professional integrity and confidentiality, but did not mention autonomy or justice. And yet they were respected.

There is a fashion for writing books which indict modern medicine.[2] The authors who write these books attack the medical profession for its precipitous use of dangerous technologies and treatments (for example diethylstilboestrol (DES), which caused vaginal sarcoma; thalidomide; and the artificial heart), for its indifference to social issues (particularly the issue of distributive justice), its self-interest in the promotion of inappropriate research, its greed, its inability to communicate with the public at large, its single-minded pursuit of science at the expense of the humane, and for its collusive inaction when faced with the fraud or malpractice of its colleagues — witness the McBride affair and the Chelmsford Hospital disaster in Australia in recent years. Dr McBride, an eminent gynaecologist and obstetrician in Sydney, Australia, is generally credited with being the first to appreciate that the drug thalidomide caused birth defects in the children of mothers who had taken the drug during pregnancy. He began a crusade to find other drugs that might have the same effect, and made claims that he had experimental evidence that implicated another drug commonly prescribed during pregnancy. Subsequently, it was alleged that he had falsified evidence from his experiments. As a result, he appeared before an inquiry, and was deregistered as a medical practitioner (see also chapter 3). At Chelmsford Hospital, Dr Harry Bailey, a prominent psychiatrist, treated patients with various psychiatric conditions by 'deep sleep therapy'. The evidence for its effectiveness was slender, and the pharmacological sleep induced could last for weeks at a time. The monitoring and documentation of the prolonged sleep state were inadequate, and there were several deaths. The profession was slow to realise what was happening. The inquiry that followed took several years, and Dr Bailey committed suicide before its adverse findings were handed down.

There is, therefore, some substance in these accusations, and the time has come for the medical profession to reflect seriously on these perceptions of failure, in the midst of their very clear successes.

Sociologists, economists, epidemiologists and politicians have all tried to show their understanding of the issues. The practice of medicine continues in the hands of clinicians who cater, at least in Westernised countries, for a belief in health as an individual right, and who continue to deliver personal services for reward. The vested interests maintaining one-to-one medicine are very strong, and they are not purely mercenary. The Hellenic–Judaeo–Christian valuation of individual human life still persists in a society which sets a diminishing value on religious belief.

It is hard for doctors and patients to communicate, and some of this difficulty arises from modern science and its somewhat uneasy place in medicine. There is little doubt that doctors and patients have failed to communicate with each other in the past, but there are now whole industries of commentary and a whole language of inadequacy which have been generated by psychologists, allied health professionals, philosophers and the medical profession itself with which to define perceived failures to communicate adequately with an increasingly literate and litigious public. The doctor-as-patient should therefore provide a useful perception of the realities and myths which underpin the overt and latent hostility expressed by the general public towards the medical profession as a whole (although relatively rarely towards 'their particular doctor').

The ill doctor ought to be able to provide insight into the experience of what it is to be ill, what it is like to lose autonomy[3] and what it is to communicate with the medical profession. Despite the common view that doctors make poor communicators, the clarity of much medical writing and speaking says otherwise. Keats,[4] Sachs,[5] Frank,[6] Zaret,[7] Rabin,[8] Rosenbaum[9] and Ingelfinger,[10] for example, have all left compelling accounts of their illnesses. The intensely objective and profoundly moving account by Ingelfinger[10] of the experience of his fatal oesophageal cancer created a considerable stir at the time, and made clinicians talk and think about the issue of their own adequacy as carers. And yet this remarkable record, left by a great physician of this generation, had no enduring effect on attitudes, paradigms and medical curricula. The inadequacies underlined by Ingelfinger were accepted as important, but not as important as the prevailing reductionist, mechanistic model of medical practice. ('Paradigms' are ways of viewing things using accepted assumptions and clear models: 'reductionist' means understanding complex theories or systems in terms of simpler concepts or their isolated components.)

There are other profound insights offered by clinicians and their families into the nature of illness and the clinical encounter.

David Rabin[8] suffered from amyotrophic lateral sclerosis. Of one of his medical experiences, he wrote:

> I travelled to a prestigious medical centre renowned for its experience with ALS. The diagnostic and technical skills of the people were superb, and more than matched the reputation of the institution. The neurologist was rigorous in his examination and deft in reaching an unequivocal diagnosis. My disappointment stemmed from his impersonal manner. He exhibited no interest in me as a person, and did not make even a perfunctory inquiry about my work . . . I still recall that the only time he seemed to come alive during our interview was when he drew the mortality curve among his collected patients for me. 'Very interesting,' he said, 'there's a break in the slope after three years.'

The frailty of the sick clinician

Not all the strain between clinician-patient and clinician-therapist is the fault of the clinician-therapist. Martha Lear[11] wrote about the attitudes of her physician-husband wrestling with cardiac disease:

> They were trained like that, to anthropomorphize disease. Some diseases were enemies you could not vanquish: terminal cancers, inexorable progressions downwards. Others were mischievous little bastards — sleepers, simple prostates and kidney stones that should have been an easy win but might put up a hell of a fight, even to death . . . It was not a thing, not a germ, not a kidney stone, not a cancer or an infection. It was simply this process which was wearing him out, filling him with pain and frustration, and he wanted to fight it aggressively, as he had been trained to do.

Nor do physicians preserve their objectivity and sense of equality with colleagues when they become patients. Rosenbaum[9] — rather to his own surprise — found himself agreeing with his therapist even when he could perceive no benefit to his muscular weakness: 'I really didn't notice any difference in the muscles, but I didn't want to hurt her feelings. That was dumb, but it is a common reaction of patients: don't upset the doctor or he or she won't like you and won't take good care of you. I was startled by that insight.' The physician Frank[6] reported a conversation with his cardiologist after his coronary occlusion:

> We talked about my heart as if we were consulting about some computer that was producing errors in the output. 'It' had a problem. Our talk was classier than the conversations that I have with the mechanic who fixes my car, but only because my doctor and I were being vague. He was not as specific as my mechanic usually is. I knew more about hearts than I know about cars, but this engine was inside me, so I was even more reluctant to hear about the scope of the damage.

Even doctors, therefore, seem to recognise failings in their colleagues which reflect an inability to communicate what modern medicine can achieve, and what it cannot. It seems that the rise of science in medicine has expanded the objective achievements of medicine, but has at the same time created a barrier to the free communication that should exist between the public and practitioners. Medicine has, in short, failed in one of its primary functions. It has failed to adapt its paradigms to changing times, and it has relied on past patterns of success to sustain its public image and justify its heavy demands on public funds.

Limits to the length of life and the cost of health

Whatever we would like to hope to the contrary, there is a limit to human life expectancy. Hayflick[12] claimed in 1977 that there is a limit to the number of divisions that human cells can make, and extrapolated from that to predict an average human life span that is unlikely to be more than 90 years. Epidemiological data suggest that an average span of between 82 and 86 years could be realised in developed countries,[13] and in the United States the average is not far short of that. ('Epidemiology' deals with the incidence and transmission of disease in populations, especially with the aim of controlling it.)

As Maloney[14] pointed out, age distributions follow different patterns in different communities. In India, taken as a model of a developing nation, the age distribution is heavily positively skewed. This is caused by a high birth rate and a high mortality from diseases which cause death at a relatively young age. By contrast, the age distribution in the developed United States is more nearly rectangular, until about the age of 70 years when there is a steady decline caused by the degenerative diseases, cancer, coronary artery disease and stroke. Maloney emphasised that about 26 years have been added to average life expectancy in the 20th century, but nothing to maximum life expectancy. He said: 'The medical task in a developed country is largely accomplished so far as longevity is concerned.' Life expectancy as a measure of medical achievement is no longer relevant in developed societies.

The concept that life is finite does not seem to have caught the public imagination. There is still a tendency to rejoice when deaths from cardiac disease decline in frequency, without a corresponding acknowledgment that some other cause of death must be increasing in frequency. If death is inevitable, so is cost restraint. Each country has a certain pool of money on which it can draw to fund enterprises which must inevitably be in competition — defence, transport, education, arts and sport as well as health. Whatever our moral judgments or our prejudices may be, these things will compete and there will be a limit to the health budget. It does not really matter how health is funded — eventually, the users pay. They may pay quite directly, as in the United States, or largely through taxation, as in Australia.

We can make some sort of a measure of the priority given to health by measuring the proportion of gross domestic product (GDP) spent on health. These figures are familiar enough. We know that in the United States, expenditure is over 13% of GDP, that in Australia it is about 7.5%, and in Britain between 4 and 5%. The significance of these figures, however, is not clear. It is possible that there is too much being spent in the United States and too little in Britain, but there is no way to measure the truth or falsity of these claims. Studies suggest that the health of populations depends remarkably little on the system of health care delivery.[15] Whatever the ideal level of expenditure may be, there are signs that various countries are reaching the limits of expenditure. Controls are tightening in the United States, where, for example, the DRG (diagnosis related grouping) system attempts to define how long patients with a given disease can spend in hospital before their insurance funds run out. In Australia, with a lower proportion of GDP committed to health, there is already overt government anxiety that expenditure may be getting out of control, and that access to such expensive technology as MRI (magnetic resonance imaging) will have to be strictly limited, at least in the public sector. Maloney[14] suggested that 12.5% of GDP may represent an absolute ceiling, a region of revolt for the population and for government.

There is an old law of development which says that the last gains are the hardest.[16] In medicine, doctors have seen an era of rapidly increasing cost-effectiveness, the growth of whole specialties and a demonstrable prolongation of life. That era is finished. Unfortunately, the growth of costs continues, so doctors have apparently entered an era of declining cost-effectiveness. This perception will probably remain if doctors and others continue to use life expectancy as the sole measure of effectiveness.

Using cancer as a model, doctors can point to real progress in the management of some types, such as Hodgkin's disease (a lymph gland cancer), testicular cancer and some of the childhood sarcomas. These spectacular advances, however, have not been matched in the treatment of such a common tumour as colonic cancer, particularly once it has metastasised to the liver. Cancer is a fearsome disease. Its conquest will continue to attract the best minds and good research grants. But its conquest will mean an increase of some other cause of death. It may be heart disease, it may be strokes, or all ideas of a 'disease free' society may be destroyed by the AIDS epidemic. If doctors are to continue to justify high levels of expenditure on medicine and

9

health, they must look again at what they are achieving, and perhaps adopt new measures of effectiveness.

Doctors are being pressed to limit costs, and much of the discussion of medicine in recent years has been dominated by its supply-side economics. To understand cost increase, it is necessary to understand the components of medical cost. The first of these might be the salaries and fees of the medical profession itself. Moore[17] pointed out that very strict control of surgical fees, involving an across-the-board reduction of 25%, would reduce the total costs of medicine in the United States by only 0.6–1.2%. Although medical fees remain a target for reformers and legislators, they are not responsible for the ballooning of the health budget. The second group of costs are the 'hotel costs' involved in hospital treatment. American figures suggest that almost one person in eight will require either hospital treatment or day care treatment each year. These costs generate almost 50% of the total. Maloney,[14] however, pointed out that the 'hotel' expenses have risen only at the same rate as the CPI.

Expenses rise in Westernised countries partly because technology is expensive. Major technology demands major capital outlay. It then requires salaries for continued management, continuing expenses for replacement and further capital outlay to update the equipment as new developments emerge. Maloney[14] showed that expenses related to new technology rise at a rate between two and four times that of the CPI. New technology is frequently defended because it shortens the diagnostic and therapeutic process, but these savings in personal time and wages are not reflected in the health and medical budgets. Savings in time simply allow more patients to occupy a given bed, so that the total cost may actually rise as the unit cost falls.

It is not surprising, therefore, that there should be governmental moves to control technology. This is already happening in Britain, New Zealand and Australia, and the placement of lithotriptors and MRI machines will be subject to strict regulation. This may seem logical and reasonable, but there are disturbing implications. Because the delivery of services expected by the public is so dependent on technology, control of technology is the first step in control of service delivery. If services are to be limited, the decision must be made by politicians. It cannot be made solely by the medical profession. The profession delivers services according to demand and the capacity of society to pay. It cannot generate a series of technologies and skills and then deny patients access to them. It is a government responsibility to decide what a country can and cannot afford. Jennett,[18] as a clinician, outlined an agenda for the control of technology, but the medical profession can only advise on matters such as effective treatment and distribution of services. It has neither the authority nor the training to implement social reform.

The first challenge facing the profession, then, may be that of coping with an increasingly limited budget. The second, and equally exacting, challenge will be to define the achievements of our time. The third challenge, the most daunting of all, will be for doctors to communicate their 20th-century roles and accomplishments. If doctors accept that life expectancy is no longer their sole measure of achievement, then they are forced to examine the impact they have on quality of life, a subject that will recur throughout this book. Improvements in quality of life have been striking in the last 20 years. For some reason, this very positive achievement has gone unsung, and the medical profession is as much to blame as anyone. Geriatric clinics, pain clinics, palliative care units and artificial hips have all contributed to a better quality of life for groups of people who once suffered from the medical profession's lack of interest.

It is, admittedly, difficult to measure achievement in this area, and there are some who deny that it is possible to quantify a quality. Quantification of quality of life has been regarded as a 'soft' area of science, the domain of sociologists and psychologists. Nevertheless, there is an abundant literature on the subject, and there are groups actively working to develop further the methodology and accuracy of measurement,[19–24] and I will say more about this in later chapters. There is a whole field of clinical research awaiting the interest of academics and clinicians alike. There is a real need to quantify achievements in the management of advanced malignancy and incurable degenerative disease. It would seem that doctors cannot significantly prolong life, but they can add significantly to the enjoyment of what remains. It is by these means that they can most strongly justify their existence and their importance as a caring profession.

It becomes important, therefore, for doctors to redefine progress. No one can deny that the money supply is shrinking. If doctors insist on defining progress by increase in life expectancy, then they cannot deny that the cost-effectiveness of the activities of the medical profession is declining. They must learn to measure quality of life and to express modern achievements in terms of improvement of quality of life. A shift of emphasis from quantity to quality can only benefit patient care and public relations. Doctors are, whether they recognise it or not, confronting their own future. They must enter that future so that they can re-establish the public perception of their essential role in the maintenance of life, to be lived at the best possible level. In order to do that, doctors must also understand what they are doing when they learn and practise medicine, and make decisions based upon what they have learnt. Doctors must also learn to communicate effectively what they know, while recognising the imperfections of their knowledge.

This chapter has examined the perceived failures of medicine in both the social and the interpersonal domains. The rest of this book examines some of these issues, and argues for a change of medical orientation from biopositivism to the biohumane. It concentrates mainly on the interpersonal domain of the doctor–patient relationship. The next chapter examines the clinical process — the steps by which a medical consultation evolves — in order to identify the critical points where communication is most likely to fail.

NOTES

1. Hafferty F, Salloway JC. The evolution of medicine as a profession. A 75 year perspective. Minnesota Medicine 1993; 76:26–35.

2. See, for example, Dutton DB. Worse than the disease: pitfalls of medical progress. Cambridge: Cambridge University Press, 1988; and Konner M. The trouble with medicine. Sydney: ABC Books, 1993. A most perceptive examination of the problems of modern medicine from a medical stance is found in Thomas L. The fragile species. New York: Collier Books, 1993.

3. Jensen UJ, Mooney G. Changing values: autonomy and paternalism in medicine and health care. In: Jensen UJ, Mooney G, eds. Changing values in medical and health care decision making. John Wiley & Sons, 1991:1–15.

4. Keats J. The life and letters of John Keats. Richardson J. London: Folio Society, 1981.

5. Sachs O. A leg to stand on. New York: Summit Books, 1984.

6. Frank AW. At the will of the body. Boston: Houghton Mifflin, 1991.

7. Zaret BL. Trauma. In: Mandell et al (eds). When doctors get sick. New York: Plenum Publishing, 1987:405–11.

8. Rabin D. Occasional notes: compounding the ordeal of ALS: isolation from my fellow physicians. New England Journal of Medicine 1982; 307:506–9.

9. Rosenbaum EE. A taste of my own medicine: when the doctor is the patient. New York: Random House, 1988.

10. Ingelfinger FJ. Arrogance. New England Journal of Medicine 1980; 303:1507–11.

11. Lear MW. Heartsounds. New York: Simon & Schuster, 1980:152.

12. Hayflick L. The cell biology of human aging. Scientific American 1980; 242:42–9.

13. Fries JF. Aging, natural death and the compression of morbidity. New England Journal of Medicine 1980; 303:130–5.

14. Maloney JV. Presidential address: the limits of medicine. Annals of Surgery 1981; 194:247–55.

15. Kohn R, White KL, eds. Health care: an international study. Report of the World Health Organisation collaborative study of medical care utilizations. London: Oxford University Press, 1976:392.

16. Landes DS. Revolution in time: clocks and the making of the modern world. Cambridge (Massachusetts) and London: Belknap Press of Harvard University Press, 1983:132.

17. Moore FD. Surgical stresses in the flow of health care financing. The role of surgery in national expenditure: what costs are controllable? Annals of Surgery 1985; 201:132–41.
18. Jennett B. High technology medicine: benefits and burdens. New York: Oxford University Press, 1986.
19. Spitzer WO, Dobson AJ, Hall J, Chesterman E, Levi J, Shepherd R, Battista RN, Catchlove BR. Measuring the quality of life of cancer patients: a concise QL-index for use by physicians. Journal of Chronic Disease 1981; 34:585–97.
20. Huskisson EC. Visual analogue scales. In R Melzuck, ed. Pain measurement and assessment. New York: Raven Press, 1983:33–7.
21. Clark A, Fallowfield LJ. Quality of life measurements in patients with malignant disease. Journal of the Royal Society of Medicine 1986; 79:165–9.
22. Little JM. A method of calculating the value of palliative care of cancer patients. Australian and New Zealand Journal of Surgery 1987; 57:393–7.
23. Melzack R. The short-form McGill pain questionnaire. Pain 1987; 30:191-7.
24. Torrance GW. Utility approach to measuring health related quality of life. Journal of Chronic Disease 1987; 40:593–600.

2

The Clinical Process: A Popperean Analysis

The clinical process[1] is complicated. It has three phases — an input, the process itself, and an output. The input represents individual patients with a perceived health problem, accompanied by an extraordinarily complex network of beliefs, prejudices, fears and pressures generated by their own education and experience, by family members and friends, by book and media-driven information, by cultural background and education and by societal attitudes towards various diseases. The output represents the medical achievement — the change in expectation and quality of life, the variation in the burden of disease, and the relief of specific symptoms. Outcomes are hard to measure. This chapter deals predominantly with the process experienced by patients who consult a doctor or a clinic, and who follow the sequence of events that are begun by the consultation. It is impossible to avoid considering the nature of the patients or the nature of their perceived illnesses or, for that matter, the influence of societal attitudes toward illness, at least briefly. So complex and important are the input and output, however, that they would need separate and lengthy discussion to do them justice.

Why discuss the consultative, investigative and therapeutic process at all? Is there a problem with a course of action which has apparently evolved slowly and appropriately over many centuries, and which is used every day by thousands of clinicians and their patients? There are, indeed, signs of discontent in both patients and doctors. Medical schools are changing their curricula because the teachers perceive deficiencies in the way that the clinical experience is communicated to students. Medical consumer groups criticise the profession for its impersonality, its poor communication of the alternatives to 'standard' treatment and its apparent self-interest. Complaints departments are among the fastest growing paramedical groups, and about 60% of complaints levelled against an Australian teaching hospital in one study[2] concerned communications or 'the system'. Malpractice insurance premiums are increasing in some countries because litigation is increasing in frequency and monetary returns, a sure sign of uneasiness in relationships between the profession and its clients. Defensive medicine is an established part of practice in some countries. Government, appalled by the cost of health, is preaching efficiency, best practice, competitive bidding and funding based on workloads for publicly funded hospitals. There may not be any direct measures of the performance of the clinical process, but there are operational measures of dissatisfaction with the clinical encounter. There seems, therefore, to be a problem. While there may not be any definitive solutions, it is worthwhile to define the problem more clearly as a starting point for tentative and trial solutions.

The Popper model

While there have been strong criticisms[3] of Karl Popper's epistemological system, the clinical encounter conforms in some ways to his model of the evolutionary approach to scientific problems.[4, 5] ('Epistemology' is the philosophical study of the nature, origins and limitations of knowledge.) The fruitfulness of employing a philosophical system — even when the system is open to serious criticism — has been demonstrated by Toombs in her detailed analysis of the meaning of illness.[6] Toombs, a philosopher who has multiple sclerosis, has used Husserl's phenomenological approach[7] to dissect the nature of the relationship of the 'ill' person to the illness and to the clinician treating the illness. (In the introduction to her book, Toombs gives a concise account of Husserl's phenomenology. Ricoeur[8] also offers a major critique of Husserl, and argues strongly for his own hermeneutic approach.)

In Popper's terminology, the scientific method can be represented in a four-step model as follows:

$$P1 \rightarrow TS1 \rightarrow EE \rightarrow P2$$

where P1 is the initial problem, TS1 the first trial solution or hypothesis, EE is the phase of error elimination in which the theory is subjected to the process of severe criticism and testing, and P2 is the residual problem remaining after the error elimination process.

In clinical terms, P1 is the presenting problem which the patient brings to the clinician; TS1 is the provisional diagnosis reached after the history and physical examination have been carried out; EE is the process of further testing — blood counts, biochemistry, endoscopy, organ imaging, pathology; and P2 is the nosological problem of classifying the disease, determining its appropriate treatment and its prognosis. ('Nosology' is the system of classifying diseases.)

Such a simple analysis is helpful only in defining the steps by which the process proceeds on a 'scientific' level. As every clinician knows, the flow is much less linear than the Popper model, largely because expression and communication are involved, and the real message of the patient may be obscured. There may be, because of fear or misinformation or misunderstanding or mis-experience on the part of the patient (the transmitter), a very high noise to signal ratio which can make interpretation of the message difficult. To compound the problem, there may be an imperfectly tuned clinician (the receiver) trying to untangle the noisy signal. The imperfect tuning may be caused by many things — innate disposition, education, cultural differences, language difficulties, personal antipathy or fatigue, to name a few. The tuning of the transmitter and of the receiver may thus be incompatible, and even a long consultation may not result in communication.

The problem of language

One of the major problems of the clinical relationship is the need for language. Medical professionals are taught at school and university that precise language is a virtue, and they tend to admire those who can express themselves clearly and concisely. They also tend to like those patients who express themselves well, and give a 'good' history, that is, a history which fits the pattern of a 'classical' story of a disease. Patients who describe abdominal pain which always starts 30 minutes after a meal, wakes them in the early hours of the morning and is relieved by alkali, have a classical history of peptic ulceration, and teachers like to introduce such people to students, reinforcing in their minds the classical — and relatively rare — model. Unfortunately, language is seldom used in a purely objective way, either by patients or doctors.

Popper,[4,5] following Buhler,[9] pointed out that everyday language exists on a number of levels. Perhaps the lowest and most primitive level is the expressive or emotional level. This level (which may be non-verbal) can be seen in many animals as well as in people. It comprises screams of pain or fear, grunts of surprise, and the laughter of pleasure. The second level is the signalling level, which appeals to the receiver for support or joint action. Once again, this may be non-verbal. It may express itself in body language by such phenomena as a dry mouth or an imploring look. It may also be verbal, expressed as something like 'It's not serious, is it?' The third level, a purely verbal level, is the descriptive, and it is the first level which sets people apart on the evolutionary scale. While it appears that bees have some capacity for description through dancing,[10] and that chimpan-

18

zees may have some capacity for synthetic language,[11] the human capacity to use words to communicate the attributes of an object or an experience is unique, and has been of incalculable survival advantage. The fourth level is the argumentative. It is a level of language that requires reciprocity so that discussion and criticism may be exchanged and enhanced. There are other forms of language, such as the hortatory and persuasive or oratorical, but these play a relatively small part in medical encounters.

In the clinical situation, clinicians and their patients may expect to deal with each other with descriptive or argumentative language — the highest and most objective levels. The problem is that levels one and two are always present as well. It is impossible to avoid altogether the expressive and signalling functions, as they are embedded in all human spoken communication. Clinicians recognise this indirectly when they describe someone who copes with bad clinical news without expression or signalling as 'handling it too well', and predict a rapid descent into depression or agitation. They recognise that they are not receiving appropriate signals, and that this is just as important as receiving a signal. We will examine the problems of language in more detail in chapter 10.

Worlds 1, 2 and 3

Is it possible to objectify problems by consciously insisting on objective language? The answer is very clearly 'No'. Not only do the patients' vulnerability and fear hamper straightforward communication, but there are also innumerable misapprehensions working on both sides of the consultation that make a straightforward exchange of information virtually impossible. (In this context, Gadamer's 'horizons of communication' and Habermas's concept of 'ideology critique' are illuminating — see chapter 10.) The Popperean model of worlds 1, 2 and 3[4,5] is of some use in examining my meaning.

In Popper's pluralistic (and much criticised[3]) model, world 1 is the world of objects, of things that have a material existence available to sense perception. World 2 is the inner world of private thoughts, experiences and beliefs, peculiar to each individual. World 3 is the world of concepts, theories and objective knowledge, including language, law, philosophy, religion, science, the arts and institutions. In Popper's view, world 3 consists of all objective knowledge, whether false or not, which has the potential to be criticised objectively. Testing cannot, according to Popper, establish whether a theory or a law or a belief is 'true'. In his philosophy, proof by induction is never valid; only falsity is undeniable, the finding of an exception to a rule. Progress results from the four-step process outlined above: the process of identifying a problem (the exception to a rule), the formulation of a new theory, the process of testing until a new error is found, and the new problem thus uncovered. The process of improvement in world 3 contents is thus endless, and dependent on constant feedback.

It is obvious that a significant part of the knowledge content of medicine (though not all of it) exists in world 3. It has been error tested in the approved way, and is available for clinicians to use in working hypotheses. The process of problem identification and error testing continues, so the working hypotheses change, but good clinicians will have a command of the best available information at the time within their special field. This does not mean that every clinician with specialist training in a particular field will reach the same nosological conclusion and advise the same treatment, given the same objectively generated data examinable in world 1 with world 3 theories and knowledge. For one thing, each clinician has different values and personal experiences, often deeply held in world 2, and never subjected to the challenge and modification that come from exposure in world 3 to discussion, publication or presentation. In addition, medical knowledge is often probabilistic. The clinician, dealing one-to-one with a sick person, cannot state the best treatment for the most likely diagnosis in that person. The clinician may know precisely the probability of a diagnosis and the likelihood of a cure with a certain treatment, but cannot know the outcome for the individual. Also, the clinician's advice will be affected by a host of subjective considerations: will the side effects be worse than the symptoms of untreated disease, will the mutilation of treatment irreparably destroy the quality of life, do these (to the clinician) minor symptoms justify a joint replacement? It is this interaction between worlds 2 and 3 that produces different advice from different clinicians, and makes second opinions so very difficult and confusing. Conflicting opinions may both be valid: they may be based on a similar assessment of the odds and probabilities, but reflect the risk-taking propensities of different individuals. There is nothing wrong with second opinions, as long as patients understand that they are nothing more than informed advice from a clinician. A sound acquaintance with the medical knowledge in world 3 does not guarantee certainty. A broad knowledge of the other contents of world 3 — art, philosophy and science — and a personal involvement with the problems of science and creativity may allow a 'wiser' conversation, but still cannot guarantee the 'right' result.

If the situation is difficult for clinicians, it is even more confusing for patients, who are experiencing illness in a personal way in world 2 but are expected to provide and discuss most of the medical information in world 1 or world 3. Pain, for example, is a personal experience, and its significance or meaning for patients begins in world 2. Yet clinicians will try to objectify symptoms, questioning patients about their attributes — severity, site, radiation, periodicity and relief. Clinicians examine the personal experience as a semi-concrete object in world 1 with criteria and rules and theories evolved in world 3. To complicate the transaction further, patients have often discussed symptoms within their own information circle, and evolved world 3 concepts and theories about their own bodily functions and disorders. These ideas may be quite false and easily falsifiable, but they are nevertheless held by patients and are part of their world 3 'knowledge' structure. The clinicians' attempts to discuss the clinical problem will use their world 3 base, which is seldom the same as the patients' world 3 base. Unless language is used very carefully, with considerable sensitivity for the inevitable clash of world 3 theories, communication will fail, simply because there has been no resolution of the world 3 differences.

One of the greatest difficulties of this world 3 communication arises, as we have seen, from the probabilistic nature of much clinical information. Popper[4] was dismissive of Bayesian methods, a mathematical model for adjusting probability values as new information becomes available, but his specific objection was in the area of subjectivist epistemology. From a practical point of view, clinical communication of the uncertainty inherent in clinical judgment must take account of probabilities. Where appropriate studies have been made, clinicians who know the literature (world 3) can say: 'You have a 75% chance of living five years with this condition and that treatment.' What they cannot say — and what patients usually want to hear — is: 'I am sure that you are one of the 75%.' Toombs,[6] speaking from the patient's perspective, says: 'The patient thus comes to the physician with the unrealistic expectation that . . . a complete restoration of health will be forthcoming. If the physician is unable to fulfil this expectation, the patient is overwhelmed by a sense of helplessness and perceives the situation to be totally and irrevocably out of control.' The clinicians' world 3 provides at best some indication of a probability, but the patients' world 2 wants a certainty. It is hardly surprising that informed consent is seldom fully informed, that patients accuse doctors of being dishonest or of prevaricating, and that doctors feel that patients and their families fail to listen to advice. The difficulties of discussing probabilities are further examined in chapter 5, and informed consent is examined in chapter 9.

In the effort to gain more world 1 information (more hard data for world 3 theories and knowledge to work on) clinicians seek material beyond the world 2 and 3 offerings of patients, even though they usually make a working diagnosis within the first minute or so of the start of the clinical encounter.[12] This involves searching for physical signs and ordering tests. Physical examination may be both specific and general, and can be both reassuring and threatening to patients. Clinicians use abnormal findings and the absence of other abnormal findings to further categorise and stage illness. They may run through a checklist of attributes of a lump — its site, size, consistency, fixity, level, tenderness, pulsatility and so on — but will be more concerned at this stage to make a broad categorisation — benign or malignant, infected or sterile, serious or trivial — rather than a precise diagnosis. Objective tests — blood counts and biochemical estimations, bacterial studies, organ imaging, biopsy studies and the like — are further extensions of the world 1 data-gathering for examination and interpretation in world 3. These tests are variably invasive, painful and threatening. Something belonging to patients is taken and submitted to an apparently impersonal and juridical process somewhere remote and authoritative. Yet the tests are not always conclusive, and commonly they do not deliver the news that patients would like to hear. Again, the patients' world 2 and the clinicians' world 3 may come into conflict. The patients seek reassurance.[6] Modern clinicians aspire to objective science, however unsuccessfully. This is the source of a tension which is nearly impossible to resolve, because it runs so deeply and is so poorly acknowledged by either patients or clinicians. It is the underlying theme of this book.

Humanism in medicine

This raises the whole question of humanism in medicine. Conventionally, humanism in medicine is equated with empathy and sympathetic understanding — the capacity to enter the world 2 of suffering patients and to share the suffering. The medical profession is accused of a lack of empathy, and there is a general feeling that scientific detachment has been taken too far in the value system of medical practitioners. Such a claim could be

endlessly and pointlessly debated, since there are only anec-
dotes, without data, to support the accusations, and there are no
standards by which to measure the empathic performance of an
entire profession. The adverse judgment is based, therefore, on
intuitive perceptions. Yet we must ask how far it is really appropriate for clinicians to try to enter the personal worlds of
suffering of their patients. The great French actor Coquelin, who
created the role of Rostand's Cyrano de Bergerac, said that
believing a stage part could only be 'lived' by entering the actual
experience of the character was the mark of amateur actors, and
that amateurs would therefore exhaust themselves within a few
performances. Professionals understood and could detach themselves from the experiences of the character, and could watch
their own performance objectively. In this way, professionals
could create the right impression night after night without the
emotional exhaustion of nightly attempts to experience the
emotions of the character.

Popper[13] expressed that view succinctly: 'I hold that it is impossible for us to love or to suffer with a great number of people;
nor does it appear to me very desirable that we should, since it
would ultimately destroy either our ability to help or the intensity of these very emotions . . . We can love mankind only in
certain concrete individuals. But by the use of thought and imagination, we may become ready to help all who need our help.'
Understanding, which is a world 3 activity, thus becomes more
important than an exhausting fellow-feeling in clinical encounters. Understanding can be equated with problem-solving, and
all participants in the clinical process seek the solution to a problem. We will examine the concept of understanding in chapter
10.

Popper[4] also had something to say about the attributes of
people who are likely to be good as problem-solvers:

> I also suggest that the much discussed problem of the transference
> of learning from one discipline to another is closely connected with
> gaining experience in wrestling with live problems. Those who have

learned only how to apply some given theoretical framework to the solving of problems . . . cannot expect that their training will help them much in another specialism. It is different with those who have themselves wrestled with problems, especially if their understanding, clarification, and formulation, proved difficult.

Clinicians who are widely read and broadly educated, who have grappled with research as part of their training and with literature, philosophy, science or anything outside their profession which taxes their understanding and intelligence, are likely to be able to identify and address the interconnecting problems in the interconnected worlds that their patients present. And they will do this better than their equally intelligent colleagues who restrict themselves intellectually to the confines of their profession. This is the strongest argument for a liberal education for medical graduates. But it is not an argument for adding strands of literature, philosophy, politics and art to medical courses which are already crammed with the necessary — if sometimes shaky — science that makes the basis of clinical practice. A compulsory course in creative writing will not produce a generation of authors. All people are not equally curious or active intellectually. Perhaps medical faculties should go much further in their search for people with a demonstrable involvement in world 3 activities before they enter medicine. It seems highly likely that the perceived inadequacies of medical graduates may reflect dissatisfaction with the restricted, trade-oriented views of modern universities and the students they select. The best-motivated teachers cannot change the motivations of students, who view medicine as a trade to be entered after mastering a body of knowledge — a view reinforced by the examination system and the didactic teaching appropriate to the examination requirements. It may be more logical to change the student population at entry by new selection criteria than to try to change inappropriate students by compulsory education in 'mind-enlarging' areas. Curious and demanding students will demand a change in teaching and a change in the performance of teachers, and their feedback will reward the change. Imposing new teaching methods and new standards for teachers cannot be guaranteed to change the attitudes of students selected largely for their capacity to pass their final school examinations with high marks. We will discuss these matters in more detail in chapter 11.

It is essential for all clinicians — whether students, experienced practitioners or those in between — to realise that the clinical process is fuzzy and messy and imprecise. Clinicians and patients may be, in Popper's terms, worlds apart, and if neither party understands why this is so the gap can only widen, and the measures of dissatisfaction will show more clearly. At the heart of the problem lies a division between the outcome of the clinical experience and the perceptions of that outcome, by patients and clinicians. Outcome for clinicians is assessed in world 1 with world 3 criteria: a gangrenous leg has been amputated; the patient's life has been saved; intolerable pain has been relieved; toxicity and confusion have gone. Of course, there has been a price: the leg has gone; and there is a level of disability which will persist for life. But there was no choice, no other treatment. So the outcome was a good one. The patients' main assessment takes place in world 2 and world 1: a major piece of the body has irreparably gone; the inability to get up to pass urine at night is undeniable and undignified; the experience of phantom pain is real but is not communicable, and is almost as distressing as the poorly remembered pain of the gangrenous leg. The patients' world 2 assessment may well be that life has changed, and that its quality has diminished.

Clinical medicine cannot always maximise satisfaction, but it can aspire to minimise dissatisfaction. Deciding what satisfaction is for someone else is potentially authoritarian.[14] Only individual patients can know what will really satisfy them. The removal of an inflamed appendix saves life and relieves pain, but at the price of a scar and adhesions. Treatment of pneumococcal pneumonia with penicillin is brilliantly successful in relieving the infection and its dangerous consequences, but takes time and may leave lung scarring. A hip replacement may relieve the pain of osteoarthritis, but hip movements do not return to 'normal'. There is a price for all medical treatment, and in that price lies the ultimate source of dissatisfaction with the clinical process.

The clinical encounter is perceived as an unpleasant necessity, but clinicians' understanding of the depth of dissatisfaction is very weak. They know that the epiphenomena of dissatisfaction — complaints, litigation, legislation, economic intervention and consumer protest — are all increasing, but they have only dim and fragmentary ideas about the nature of the problem. The problem must be defined and understood if doctors are to improve their performance and the public perception of that performance. Their major weakness is an unwillingness to respond to feedback from those dissatisfied with the clinical experience. Doctors treasure the positive reports that they get from grateful patients, the letters and presents, the cards carefully displayed in the hospital entrance lobby. But approval cannot tell them how to improve: it can only confirm what is perceived as 'right' about the clinical process. It cannot tell doctors what needs to be reformed. Culturally, doctors are attuned to regard a complaint as a threat. The natural response is to become defensive, to cover tracks and to find reasons to say that the complainant is wrong. Thus doctors lose an opportunity to define the elusive problems that make for dissatisfaction. Until they learn that complaints are an opportunity to examine and evaluate their performance — perhaps the only really worthwhile opportunity[15] — they will go on the way they are, and the gap between the profession and the increasingly informed public will increase.

There are signs that patients are often dissatisfied with the clinical encounter. Medical curricula are changing, medical consumer groups ask to be heard and litigation adds to the cost of medicine in some countries. Popper's views on the nature and progress of science provide some helpful insights into the nature of the clinical process and its problems. In particular, his theory of the process and progress of science, his views on language and communication and his theory of worlds 1, 2 and 3 can all be applied to the transactions between doctors and patients. The need for humanism in medicine is supported by this analysis, as is a mechanism to allow feedback of criticism from patients to the medical profession, so that the profession can review its performance continually. It is also evident that clinicians need to understand in more detail what happens as patients and doctors communicate, when the one side gives and the other takes the medical history. That is the subject of chapter 10. Before we examine that transaction, we need to understand the process by which medicine generates the knowledge that it uses — the contents of Popper's world 3.

NOTES

1. Much of the material in this chapter originally appeared in The problem of the clinical process — a Popperean analysis. Theoretical Surgery 1993; 8:146–150. It is reproduced with the kind permission of the editors.
2. Little JM. Enantiology as a tool for decision making about patient satisfaction (abstract). Theoretical Surgery 1992; 7:153–4.
3. Tiles M. Method and the authority of science. In: Griffiths AP, ed. Key themes in philosophy. Cambridge: Cambridge University Press, 1989:31–51.
4. Popper KR. Objective knowledge: an evolutionary approach. Oxford: Clarendon Press, 1979.
5. Popper KR. Conjectures and refutations: the growth of scientific knowledge. London and New York: Routledge, 1989.
6. Toombs SK. The meaning of illness: a phenomenological account of the different perspectives of physician and patient. Dordrecht: Kluwer Academic Publishers, 1992.
7. Husserl E. Ideas: general introduction to pure phenomenology, Gibson WRB, trans. London: Collier Books, 1969.
8. Ricoeur P. From text to action. Illinois: Northwestern University Press, 1991.
9. Bühler K. Die geistege entwicklung des kindes, 2nd edn. Jena: Fischer, 1921. Cited in Popper KR. Objective knowledge: an evolutionary approach. Oxford: Clarendon Press, 1979:235; Popper KR. Conjectures and refutations: the growth of scientific knowledge. London and New York: Routledge, 1989:295.

10. Frisch K von. The dancing bees: an account of the life and senses of the honey bee, 2nd edn, Isle D, Walker N, trans. London: Methuen, 1966.
11. Lyons J. Chomsky, London: Fontana Press, 1991:140–5.
12. Wilbush J. The Sherlock Holmes paradigm — detectives and diagnosis. Discussion paper. Journal of the Royal Society of Medicine 1992; 85:342–5.
13. Popper KR. The open society and its enemies, vol II: the high tide of prophecy. New Jersey: Princeton University Press, 1971:240.
14. Jensen UJ, Mooney G. Changing values: autonomy and paternalism in medicine and health care. In Jensen UJ, Mooney G, eds. Changing values in medical and health care decision making. John Wiley & Sons, 1990.
15. Little JM. Decisions in clinical management: a case scenario. Medical Journal of Australia 1993; 158:204–7.

3

Science and the Epistemology of Clinical Medicine

Epistemology is that branch of philosophy which deals with knowledge, attempting to answer the basic questions 'What do we know?' and 'How do we know it?' It questions the mechanisms by which we acquire knowledge and the degree of certainty that we attach to the knowledge that we gain. Very broadly, there has been a debate between two schools of thought since the time of Plato. Rationalists, such as Plato and Descartes, contend that knowledge is intrinsic to ideas of reason solely within the mind. Empiricists insist that knowledge has no other derivation than sense experience. There has been a similar debate between realists, who insist that physical objects exist whether they are perceived or not, and idealists who contend that the external world is in some way a creation of the perceiving mind. Materialists contend that everything that exists, including abstractions like mind and colour, consists of matter or exists entirely because of material structure. Dualists hold that there is a distinction to be drawn between mind and material body. Positivists believe that all knowledge is contained within science, and that ethical, spiritual and religious speculations are to be dismissed as fruitless. We will not deal in any depth with these concepts, which are discussed in basic philosophical texts.[1-3] It is sufficient to say that Western medicine has evolved very strongly in the traditions of empiricism, realism, materialism and positivism. For these reasons, the scientific or experimental method is highly valued by medical scientists.

The experimental method and value judgments

What is understood by the term 'experimental method' (which is usually taken to have the same meaning as the scientific method) in the physical sciences? Stebbing[4] examined the experimental method in detail, and produced the following description of its paradigm:
1. formulation of a question in specific terms;
2. definition of the constituent factors of the complex situation;
3. definition of factors to be controlled;
4. controlled variation of factors one at a time;
5. wide variation of supposedly irrelevant factors in order to confirm their irrelevance;
6. avoidance of the introduction of new factors which may influence the outcome.

Stebbing said that 'These rules may be summed up in the formula: Analysis of the given situation and control of the conditions so that every relevant factor can be varied one at a time are the essential preconditions of scientific experimental investigations.' These conditions can be met in some laboratory investigations, but human variation and the inability to achieve total 'control' of variables make the criteria too stringent for most medical — particularly clinical — research. The classical statistical tests for difference or association were developed for the kinds of data that can be scrupulously controlled. The social sciences — if they are strictly sciences — have developed statistical methods that are better able to handle the data from clinical investigations.

31

What does science do?

Scientific research aims to achieve at least three ends: classification, explanation and the elucidation of cause. Classification is fundamental to science. It allows phenomena to be grouped in a way that makes their formal understanding easier and more meaningful. The Linnean system has served zoologists well, while the nosological (disease classification) system of medicine allows practitioners to recognise groups of diseases with common features and to distinguish among them those that will respond to different treatments. The classification of the lymphomas illustrates how well this system works, since it determines a standard diagnostic terminology, provides guides to the appropriate treatment of each diagnostic entity and allows broad prognostic judgments.[5]

Explanation is one of the fundamental roles of scientific endeavour, but its analysis is complex, and philosophers disagree over details. Hempel[6] described two explanatory models, the deductive–nomological and the probabilistic. The deductive-nomological model is the one familiar to schoolchildren studying Euclidean geometry. A covering law and a series of auxiliary statements culminate in an inevitable conclusion, a deductively valid statement reached by way of a series of true premises. In medicine, numbness in the distribution of an injured nerve may be explained by saying:

1. intact nerves convey sensations to the brain which may be felt as touch, temperature, vibration or pain;
2. these sensations can only get back to the brain through the peripheral nerves;
3. the anterior cutaneous nerve of the thigh in this individual has been cut across;
4. therefore, this person cannot feel touch, temperature, vibration or pain in the distribution of that nerve.

The deductive–nomological explanation is considered to be the most powerful explanatory process because of its deductive validity.

Unfortunately, deductive–nomological explanations are not uniformly available in clinical medicine, which has a basically probabilistic epistemological base. Clinicians' knowledge is empirically based, and their clinical 'laws' are inductively derived, and can never be completely secure. From experience, physicians may reason inductively that all patients with fully developed AIDS will die within a circumscribed time, because that is what has happened so far. But there is no mathematical model or basic physical law which says that future patients with developed AIDS will not overcome the illness because of a change in the virus or a mutation in the patients' genetic maps, or even because of developments that cannot be foreseen with the present knowledge base. The probability of death may be very high, but there is no natural law comparable to the laws of gravitation or universal relativity which makes the outcome inevitable. Such a qualification applies even more strikingly when surgeons treat a colonic cancer, for example. They may say that the person with a Dukes B cancer has a 34% chance of being free of disease five years from the day of operation, but they cannot say whether that person is one of the favoured 34% or not. Inductive inference needs always to be expressed in probabilistic terms by degrees of confidence. A great deal of clinical research is designed to reclassify patients and their disease states in a way that better defines the outcomes to be expected from appropriate treatment. Again, the classification and reclassification of the lymphomas provides a good illustration of this principle. Despite the elaboration of diagnosis, however, physicians cannot guarantee cure, because the classification is empirically derived and the rates of cure are inductively inferred. They are not underpinned by a mathematical or physical model.

The problems of causation are even more complex. Aristotle[7] recognised formal, material, efficient and final causes for any happening, but this has never been regarded as a fully satisfactory account of cause. Hume[8] questioned the whole concept of causation, and suggested that the notion of cause is imposed by the human mind in order to make sense of events that are regularly conjoined in time. Mill[9] reasoned that any event was the product of a chain of prior causes. Carnap[10] concluded that a causal relationship could only be said to exist if the caused event could be logically deduced from a set of laws. The conclusion that cause is no more than a logical relationship has seemed unsatisfactory to many, and recent attempts to understand the problems have concentrated on the concept of causal networks.[11] This concept suggests that any event can be seen as the outcome of a whole network of interactions. Notions of causation in medicine have been well reviewed by Velanovich.[12] Medical notions are often naive, and there is a lingering tendency within the profession to believe that complex end-points, such as cancer, have a single cause. This view certainly dominates lay thinking, and has been reinforced in medical education by slogans such as 'No acid, no peptic ulcer'.

Is there a medical science?

There is a real question about the existence of such a thing as medical science. Hayek[13] insisted that 'science' deals with objective data and the relationships between the elements of that data. The 'social sciences' deal with relationships between humans and the relationship of humans to structures and objects, and in this sense they are subjective and therefore not 'real' sciences. If objectivity is accepted as a demarcation criterion, it would seem that much medical 'science' is not real science. Measuring levels of cytochrome P450 in chronic liver disease represents objective science in that it seeks to determine the relationship between two objectively measured things. An investigation of the quality of life of those who suffer from chronic liver disease inevitably relies on subjective criteria, and attempts to bring classical science to bear on such an analysis would be condemned as 'scientism' by Hayek, where scientism is defined as an insecurely based belief that the methods of the natural sciences can be applied to the social sciences. Furthermore, rather than a binary division between objective and subjective criteria, there may be a continuity between the poles in medical science. A study of metastatic liver cancer may contain actuarial analyses of survival data and a quality of life study. The total picture of the condition therefore contains objective and subjective data, both of which contribute to the message of the study. Medical scientists should not abandon the search for ways of measuring such concepts as quality of life; indeed, there is some evidence that such measurements compare well on a number of parameters with the more familiar laboratory measurements that scientists trust implicitly.[14]

There is room, however, for legitimate disputes about value-laden matters in such a field, and for an acceptance that different solutions may suit different societies. While social differences persist, it would be unreasonable to expect universal application for each 'solution': the concept of the 'best' treatment for a given condition is likely to remain a relative matter. This relativism may be seen by purists as distinguishing between the science of medicine and its sociology. At the same time, there is reason to accept that the sociology of medicine is every bit as important as its science, and that some parts of it can be studied by numerical methods. The science and the sociology are interwoven in the fabric of medical thought and medical epistemology. Reductionist medical science has made remarkable advances, but at the cost of its roots in the concern for the individual and social well-being of its clients. Wittgenstein[15] warned that 'The existence of the experimental method makes us think we have the means of solving the problems which trouble us; though problem and method pass one another by.'

There is clearly considerable uncertainty about the nature of science and its methods, not least in the field of medicine. Is science merely that which is done by scientists? Tiles[2] may well be right when she finds that the claims of science to a method of its own are not defensible. Is there the sharp distinction between subjective and objective data that Hayek[13] would have us believe? After all, an investigation is only undertaken because investigators have reason to engage with its central problem. It would be wrong to think that scientists work entirely objectively. They have certain beliefs which cause them to be related to the object of study.

Science in medicine is, however, generally equated with the objective science defined by Hayek. For this reason, granting bodies which give money for medical research favour projects which are designed to measure relationships between and functions of structures which can be externally evaluated, rather than relationships involving human judgment and values. This adds to the alienation between the central function of medicine — the restoration of health and welfare to individuals — and the depersonalised, mechanistic and reductionist view of 'good' science. It is time for medical scientists to reassess their priorities. The current intrusion of politicians and economists into medicine has made it clear that medical scientists' knowledge of outcomes and of the elementary behaviour of humans with diseases is singularly weak, despite their intricate knowledge of the biochemistry of disease and their advanced capacity to investigate objectively the structure and functions of the human body — skills which are the result of reductionism.

Reductionism and holism

Reductionism is the process of seeking ever more basic explanations for phenomena, and it has been immensely successful in taking medicine from its quasi-religious and often intuitive base, towards a conventionally scientific one. The biopositivist model, which is the prevailing model of health and disease in Western medicine, is essentially realistic and reductionist, but the reduction seems to operate at several levels. Oppenheim and Putnam[16] devised a system of reductive categories which, they felt, depicted six levels at which science might be carried out (see Figure 3.1).

Each level in this schema includes all higher levels. Thus, the phenomena in level 6 can be explained by mechanisms at level 5,

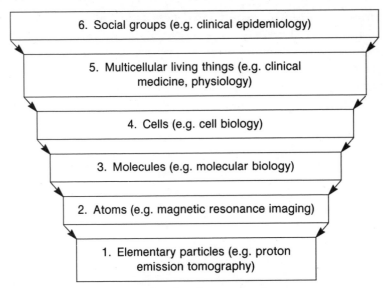

Figure 3.1 A system of reductive categories

those in level 5 by the mechanisms in level 4, and so on. The mechanisms of level 1 should then be able to explain those at all other levels. The last 40 years or so have seen a progressive reduction from the whole person with an illness (which is the fundamental unit of clinical medicine) to cellular and molecular biology as the preferred level for scientific medical research. Reductionism has as its ultimate goal the unification of all science within a single discipline, presumably that of particle physics. As Kuhn[17] pointed out, the success of any reductionist science makes the communication of its content and achievement to non-scientists progressively more difficult. This is particularly unfortunate in medicine, since communication and understanding are essential to the medical transaction.

Fodor[18] and Garfinkel[19] offered strong critiques of reductionism and the concept of the unity of all science. Holism is the opposite of reductionism. Holistic models of science are either ontological or epistemological. The ontological model insists that the complex whole is more than the sum of its parts. This implies that human health and illness cannot be satisfactorily reduced to cellular and molecular components without losing essential understanding of the impact on the whole organism. The epistemological model proposes that scientists can only test related groups of beliefs, and that testing theories in isolation from related theories cannot provide evidence for the validity of the isolated theory. The isolation process introduces a change which modifies the performance of a mechanism that functions in concert with many other mechanisms. Humanity is an irretrievably stochastic system, in this view, and the deterministic basis of reductionism is an inappropriate way to approach human well-being and its failings.

Science and medical research

Some aspects of medical research are perhaps becoming easier to understand and to define. Medical science probably does not exist in its own right. Indeed, Canguilhem[20] said that medicine seems to be 'like a technique or art at the crossroads of several sciences, rather than, strictly speaking, like one science'. Furthermore, medical science suffers from the lack of a coherent theory. The origins of medicine were holistic; its latest advances are reductionist. Some of the greatest advances in securing community welfare have followed quasi-political decisions — vaccination, sewerage, clean water supplies. The late 20th century has witnessed the triumph of technology at both the macroscopic and the microscopic levels. But those who feel that health issues are important have trouble communicating their holistic principles to scientists working within the strictly reductionist biopositivist model. So within the same discipline there are research programs that use holism, and programs that use reductionism. The most coherent and 'scientific' theories belong to the reductionists, and for this reason their programs are seen to be progressive. The holistic and reductionist schools have difficulty in communicating. Their respective paradigms can be said to be incommensurable (a term which implies that the adherents of competing theories cannot settle their differences because they do not share enough objective reference points), and in Kuhn's terms this presumably indicates the potential breakdown of the present paradigms and the start of a revolution in medical science.[17] It is possible that a unified science may emerge, but its pattern is far from clear.

Even though reductionism and the concept of a unified science may prove to be illusory, the Oppenheim–Putnam[16] stratification of levels of scientific practice is helpful in examining what research workers in medicine are actually doing. Medical research generally functions at level 3 and above, and most researchers are content to work at their chosen level without needing to understand how philosophers characterise what they are doing. Clinical epidemiologists will work at level 6, clinicians at level 5, cell biologists at level 4, molecular biologists at levels 3 and 2. Few purely medical scientists are involved in research on fundamental particles. Research at each level is essential in medicine, with its central need to apply science to classification, diagnosis, prognosis and treatment. Indeed, outcomes research at levels 5 and 6 is needed just as much as research at levels 2 and 3. Medical knowledge of outcomes is remarkably incomplete, particularly when the outcome is best expressed by measurements of quality of life. The clinical controlled trial is generally regarded by clinical scientists as the best available technique for settling questions about the outcomes of alternative forms of treatment.

The controlled trial

It is worthwhile examining briefly the concept of the controlled trial in clinical medicine. Awareness that research in medicine commonly did not meet the strong criteria of proof demanded by the natural sciences led investigators to seek powerful statistical techniques which would establish degrees of confidence for the conclusions of empirical studies. The formal process of stating a hypothesis and a null hypothesis (a detached assumption that there is no difference between treatments unless mathematics suggests otherwise when the results of the trial are statistically examined), defining conditions of entry to a trial, choosing levels of significance for statistical differences, and choosing methods of randomisation for treatment and control arms of the study, methods of blinding investigators and subjects to the nature of the treatment or placebo, and the content of the information needed to obtain informed consent, are all essential components of the controlled trial familiar to readers of the clinical research literature. The controlled trial has been the gold standard of clinical scientific performance for 50 years. But its problems are very great.

Many of the techniques of the controlled trial were not devised for medicine, but for agriculture.[21] Latin square designs (in which plots of land are divided into a grid of squares, which are randomly treated with appropriate substances in order to determine what soil additives will boost growth most effectively), the t-test (a powerful way to determine whether the average values observed in the experimental group are significantly different from those in the control group), chi-square and analysis of variance (powerful tests to detect differences between results obtained experimentally in any number of comparable groups) were designed for experiments with fertilisers and trace elements within the same or adjacent blocks of land. Similar controls are almost impossible to achieve in medicine. Crossover trials are the closest approximations that medical investigations can achieve to the neighbouring plot design. The immense artificiality of the controlled trial can be gauged by the need to distinguish efficacy from effectiveness when considering the value of a drug in therapeutics. Efficacy records the performance of the treatment under the constraints of the trial; effectiveness records the performance of the treatment in the real world of doctor–patient consultations. In addition, the Hawthorne effect[22] recognises that even beginning a study changes the outcome of the condition studied, probably because of the greater care and interest shown by the research team.

There are other problems with the controlled trial. It is costly because of the need for extra staff to accumulate the comprehensive data, and because of the common need to extend the trial to multiple institutions to recruit enough patients who satisfy the rigid entry protocols. Many trials — such as those designed to screen populations for high cholesterol levels and to lower the levels by whatever means seem appropriate — use intermediate outcomes as their end-points.[23] They are not designed to follow the studied group for life to see whether lowering cholesterol will prolong life; they use instead something that can be quickly measured, such as the levels of cholesterol before and after intervention. The true end-point is too far in the future, and can usually be expressed only in probabilistic terms. Just as the social milieu of the scientific community determines the way that science is carried out and presented, so the grant-giving process determines the life of a project and the end-points that will be used. Granting bodies cannot fund very long-term projects without committing money that might be otherwise available for other promising investigations.

The impact of ethical thinking

There are also major ethical problems that add to the problems of tightly controlled trials in medicine, problems which (rather surprisingly) have been defined clearly only in recent years. These ethical issues predominantly concern research carried out at levels 5 and 6 of the Oppenheim and Putnam schema[16] — research that concerns societies and live animals, whether human or not. The ethical movement in medicine has done much to improve the discourse on the morality of medical investigation, and it has produced stringent guidelines with which investigators should comply. A more detailed examination of ethics in medicine follows in chapters 7 and 8. It is enough to say here that in most countries no medical research can be undertaken without ethical review.

There are thus three factors which bear on the future of medical research, and which are closely and intricately connected: the biopositivist 'scientific' model of health and disease, the ethical constraints and the relative decline in available funding. The biopositivist model is powerful, but its power and the complexity of its scientific base stand in the way of easy and effective communication with those who are ill. The biopositivist model is challenged by the holistic and stochastic nature of humanity, and the controlled trial is in many ways far removed from clinical reality. The ethics of human and animal experimentation are now seen to limit the scope of whole creature research, and the issues of informed consent and animal rights are particularly contentious. Finally, the realisation that there is a finite amount of money available for all the constituents of medicine must bring about a change in approach toward research and the type of research that can be honestly justified. Medicine has diverged from the needs of its client base, and research has produced a deluge of information which is impossible to assimilate. Information is not knowledge until it can be assimilated under covering laws and applied to order the past and the future. Arndt[24] estimated that 34 000 references are added to Medline each month from 4 000 journals, and that the number of scientific journals published world-wide has passed the 100 000 mark. It is conceptually difficult to justify the generation of such a quantity of information without a plan to handle it and make sense of it.

Quantity, quality and outright fraud

The unassimilable quantity of medical publications is complemented by concerns about the quality of many papers. Lock[25] considered that only about 1% of medical publications represent 'good' science. Beyond the question of quality, there is the matter of fraud, which has been extensively discussed in the last 10 years or so. Broad and Wade[26] in 1983 examined scientific fraud generally, pointing out that Mendel's plant-breeding program produced evidence for his genetic theories of inheritance that fitted the theory too perfectly. There was evidence, they felt, that classification of characteristics had been 'massaged' to support the theory where there was any threat that the empirical findings might diverge from what had been predicted. In one sense, this does not matter, because the theory was basically correct. The claims made by Sir Cyril Burt, on the other hand, that his studies of separated twins confirmed the hypothesis that intelligence was largely inherited, were frankly misleading, and led to a serious misunderstanding of the role of environment. They were accepted without great scrutiny because they confirmed the claims made by others in the IQ movement, who discerned racial differences which they assumed to be genetic and irremediable. Burt's results were believed to be what Medawar[27] called 'lengthy and studied scientific frauds', although there is now evidence that the work was less flawed than Burt's detractors have claimed.

Medical scientific fraud began to emerge in the 1970s as a small but worrying problem. In 1974, the systematic fraud of Dr William T. Summerlin of the Sloane-Kettering Institute in New York was made public by Dr Robert Good, the supervisor of the program in which Dr Summerlin had worked. The details can be found in a 1976 article by Medawar.[28] Summerlin falsified the results of immunological experiments involving transfer of skin grafts from one mouse to another. He claimed that acceptance of a graft which should normally have been rejected rapidly could be achieved simply by maintaining the donor skin in tissue culture medium for days to weeks. This work seemed to be potentially important, not so much for any biological insight it might offer as for its potential application to human burns. The ability to harvest skin from unburnt donors, preserve it in simple tissue culture medium for long enough, and then use the skin to cover massive raw areas in patients with major burns, would have represented a significant advance in burn care. Unfortunately, the Summerlin results were faked. Skin grafts were coloured with a felt pen before photography, so that it seemed that a white mouse had accepted skin from one that was dark-skinned. Elsewhere, Medawar[29] stated that episodes of this kind would happen again, because of the immense importance of 'confidence as a bonding agent in civilisation, as it is indeed throughout professional life. Do not lawyers, bankers, clergymen. librarians, and editors tend to believe their fellow professionals unless they have good reason to do otherwise? Scientists are the same.'

The McBride case in Australia illustrates the nature of the problem. It was mentioned in Chapter 1. Credited with the first observation that thalidomide caused birth defects, Dr McBride gained an international reputation as a clinician, a scientist and crusader for scrupulous testing of the potential of new drugs to cause birth defects. Other 'discoveries' followed, and experimental work seemed to confirm his claim that at least one other drug quite commonly taken during pregnancy was also likely to interfere with foetal development. Years later, these experiments were discredited, and some of the data shown to have been falsified — although it is only fair to add that McBride has subsequently sought to justify his actions in his autobiography.

A more subtle form of falsification was examined by Medawar in 1964.[30] In a paper with the provocative title 'Is the scientific paper a fraud?', Medawar made the serious point that the conventional organisation of a scientific paper misleads the public into believing that science is logical and linear in its progress. According to the scientific paper, a scientific investigation begins with the formulation of the problem. Experiments are designed, which may resolve all or part of the problem. They are then performed, the results are analysed systematically, and a theory is formulated to explain the results. Medawar argued that most investigations begin with the theory and end with further support for it or results which do not support it. Scientists do not in fact approach their problem with an unprejudiced mind, but usually with a working hypothesis which has implications that can be tested. There are also likely to be a variety of false starts, technical problems and false trails encountered during the experiments, which will not be mentioned in the final paper.

Medawar may have been taking an extreme view for the sake of establishing an argument against the role of induction in science, but he was right in suggesting that the organisation of a scientific paper actually discourages the average reader from critical appraisal. By eliminating the weaknesses and emphasising the logical cohesion of a selected part of the experiment, scientists try to avoid contentious issues that may undermine the central thesis, and might encourage other workers to think about alternative explanations and competing hypotheses. The scientific paper may represent an essential step in the process by which science makes sense of what it does, but it may also have a negative and inhibitory effect. Graduating doctors needs to take with them the habit of continuing self-education and a developed capacity to assess the quality of the information that comes their way.

The future of medical research

All these forces combine to suggest the need for a new approach to medical, and more specifically clinical, research. There would be at least seven components in this new 'science'.

1. *Informatics*[31] is the burgeoning study of information theory and handling.
2. *Decision theory*[32] deals with making the best decision based on partial and usually probabilistic information, reflecting the reality of medical practice and clinical research.
3. *Technology assessment*[33] and *clinical epidemiology*[34] both develop an interface between informatics, decision theory and economics.

5. *Outcome research*[35] seeks ways to express the value of preventive or therapeutic medical intervention. It deals with quality of life, measures of disability and their costs, as well as the more familiar measures, such as five-year survival.
6. *Meta-analysis*[36] is a technique for the re-examination of conflicting published results in order to make a statistically valid inference from published data.
7. *Bayesian methods*[37] allow the progressive refinement of probabilistic information as more information becomes available from continued studies. Bayesian probabilities and the results of meta-analysis provide the raw material for decision-making and for technology assessment.

All these disciplines can combine to make sense of information and to provide a more secure base for practical decisions. In other words, they comprise the rational grounds for translating information into action.

Skrabanek[38] dealt harshly with risk-factor epidemiology, which is clearly a part of this process, and Little[39] offered criticisms of some of the assumptions of decision theory and technology assessment. Nevertheless, there is a growing appreciation that these techniques — which are relatively cheap to use — make maximum use of the existing data in ways which are relevant to the real world of health and illness, and that have meaning to patients, doctors, administrators, economists and politicians. Each of these groups is taking its first steps along this new pathway, which represents a recognition that good and useful science can be done within medicine at higher, more holistic levels than the conventional cellular, molecular and atomic levels. It may be a long time, however, before those who dominate research within the profession change their deeply-held view that reductionist science is the only reputable endeavour for those who want to secure their place in the honour roll of medical research. There are also definite limits to what might be achieved by even the most sophisticated and enlightened use of statistics and decision theory. Some of these shortcomings will be discussed in later chapters.

The next chapter examines the part played by authority in medicine and medical research, and the ways in which established authority moulds and perpetuates the current intellectual models of health and disease.

NOTES

1. Russell B. History of western philosophy. London: George Allen & Unwin, 1961.
2. Joad CEM. Guide to philosophy. New York: Dover Publications, 1957.
3. Passmore J. A hundred years of philosophy. Harmondsworth: Penguin, 1968.
4. Stebbing LS. A modern introduction to logic. London: Methuen, 1950.
5. Callender S, Vanhegan RI. The lymphomas. In Wetherall DJ, Ledingham JGG, Warrell DA, Oxford textbook of medicine. Oxford: Oxford University Press, 1983:160–74.
6. Hempel CG. Philosophy of natural science. Englewood Cliffs, New Jersey: Prentice-Hall, 1966: 47–69.
7. Aristotle. Quoted in: Speake J, ed. A dictionary of philosophy. London. Pan, 1979.
8. Hume D. An enquiry concerning human understanding. Selby-Bigge LA, ed. Oxford: Clarendon Press, 1991.
9. Mill JS. System of logic. London: Longman, 1961.
10. Carnap R. An introduction to the philosophy of science. New York: Basic Books, 1966.
11. Hilden J. Causal networks, not clinical trials, as a model for experimental shock research. Theoretical Surgery 1989; 4:100–2.
12. Velanovich V. Causal concepts in surgery. Theoretical Surgery 1992; 7:197–200.
13. Hayek FA. The counter-revolution of science: studies on the abuse of reason. Indianapolis: Liberty Press, 1979.
14. Wood-Dauphinée S, Troidl H. Endpoints for clinical studies: conventional and innovative variables; in Troidl H, Spitzer WO, McPeek B et al, eds. Principles and practice of research: Strategies for surgical investigators. New York: Springer-Verlag, 1991:151–68.
15. Wittgenstein L. Philosophical investigations. Oxford: Basil Blackwell, 1991.

16. Oppenheim P, Putnam H. Unity of science as a working hypothesis. In: Feigl H, Scriven M, Maxwell G, eds. Minnesota studies in the philosophy of science, vol. II. University of Minnesota Press, 1958:3–36.

17. Kuhn TS. The structure of scientific revolutions, 2nd edn. Chicago: University of Chicago Press, 1970.

18. Fodor J. Special sciences, or the disunity of science as a working hypothesis. Synthese 1974; 28:77–115.

19. Garfinkel A. Forms of explanation. New Haven: Yale University Press, 1981:49–74.

20. Canguilhem G. Ideology and rationality in the history of the life sciences, Goldhammer A, trans. Cambridge, Massachusetts: MIT Press, 1988:41–50.

21. Armitage P, Berry G. Statistical methods in medical research, 2nd edn. Oxford: Blackwell Scientific Publications, 1987:239.

22. Lyons B. Organizations. In: Heap SH, Hollis M, Lyons B, Sugden R, Weale A. The theory of choice: a critical appraisal. Oxford: Blackwell, 1994:167–8.

23. Eddy DM. Medicine, money and mathematics. American College of Surgeons Bulletin 1992; 77:36–49.

24. Arndt KA. Information excess in medicine; overview, relevance to dermatology, and strategies for coping. Archives of Dermatology 1992; 128:1249–56.

25. Lock S. Introduction. In: Lock S, ed. The future of medical journals. British Medical Journal, 1991:1–8.

26. Broad W, Wade N. Betrayers of truth: fraud and deceit in the halls of science. Century Books, 1983.

27. Medawar P. The threat and the glory: Reflections on science and scientists. Oxford: Oxford University Press, 1991.

28. Medawar P. The strange case of the spotted mice: review of Joseph Hixson, The patchwork mouse (Anchor Press, 1976). New York Review of Books, 15 April 1976.

29. Medawar P. Scientific fraud: review of W Broad and N Wade. Betrayers of truth: fraud and deceit in the halls of science (Century, 1983). London Review of Books, 17–30 November 1983.

30. Medawar P. Is the scientific paper a fraud? Saturday Review 1964 (August 1): 43–4.

31. Rootenberg JD. Information technologies in US medical schools: clinical practices outpace academic applications. Journal of the American Medical Association 1992: 268:3106–7.

32. de Dombal T, Barnes S, Dallos V et al. How should computer-aided decision support systems present their predictions to the practising surgeon? Theoretical Surgery 1992; 7:111–16.

33. Netherlands Commission on Future Health Technology. Anticipating and assessing health care technology. Dordrecht: Martinus Nijhoff Publishers, 1987.
34. Lilienfield DE. Definitions of epidemiology. American Journal of Epidemiology 1978; 107:87–90.
35. Bullinger M. Quality of life: definition, conceptualization and implications — a methodologist's view. Theoretical Surgery 1991; 6:153–48.
36. Dawson-Saunders B, Trapp RG. Basic and clinical biostatistics. Sydney: Prentice-Hall, 1990:222–4.
37. Spiegelhalter DJ, Knill-Jones RP. Statistical and knowledge-based approaches to clinical decision-support systems, with an application to gastroenterology. Journal of the Royal Statistical Society 1984; 147:35–76.
38. Skrabanek P. Risk-factor epidemiology: science or non-science? In: Health, lifestyle and environment: countering the panic. Manhattan, Manhattan Institute, 1991:47–56.
39. Little JM. Eupompus gave splendour to art by numbers. Lancet 1993; 341:878–80.

4

The Impact of Authority in Medicine and Medical Research

There can be little doubt that there is a significantly social element to science. Regardless of the strength or weakness of the various theories of science, the social impact of a period of research is very strong. A successful stint of scientific endeavour leaves young doctors with a strong sense of collegial pleasure, whatever they may feel about the existence of true science in medicine. It also produces a life-long critical attitude to evidence, and gives graduates a lasting sense of identity with the program and its director. It confers status, and defines an area of expected expertise. Most of these effects depend on the perceived authority of the research director, and that perception is determined to a great extent by the track record of the director and the productivity of the research program. Track record is judged by the director's peers and competitors, and measured scientometrically by publication numbers and quality, the number of grants obtained and the number of co-workers and research students attracted to the program. It is generally a conservative judgment, tending to perpetuate the type of science and the type of puzzle-solving condoned by the prevailing view of science within medicine.

Kitcher[1] provided a useful analysis of authority in science. Authority is either earned or unearned. Earned authority depends on track record. Unearned authority attaches to individuals because of the eminence of their teacher, or because of the eminence of the institution where they work. The dicta of an authority are often accepted as 'true', and this simplifies the process and the time-scale of learning. As Kitcher said: 'The typical scientist judges that a potential authority is sufficiently trustworthy and that acquiring the information directly would be too time-consuming.' The existence of an authority within an institution does much to enhance the collegial and mystery aspects of the social aspects of science. People who have worked at a great institution share an experience and an identity which they feel set them apart from their fellows.

But there are also negative aspects of authority. Kitcher devised a calculus for assessing authority, and drew attention to the problem of axis-splitting which may occur when authorities disagree. Undue weight given to authority may lead to excessive conservatism or to hesitation in spending time and money on replicating a crucial experiment. Pons and Fleischmann's claim[2] to have achieved cold fusion by simple means caused scientific consternation because both were well-known electrochemists, whose credentials were established. Physicists were sceptical, but the authority possessed by the authors in another branch of science meant that their work attracted attention. An established director with a major reputation and a distinguished publication record may run a degenerate program,[3] which has stopped predicting novel phenomena and which will not provide the enlarging experience anticipated by senior members of the profession and their proteges. A director whose technology has been superseded must either adapt, or continue with a degenerate program. The advent of laparoscopic surgery, for example, will profoundly affect surgical training and research programs, not simply because of changes in technique, but because of the differences in metabolic response of patients undergoing so-called minimally invasive surgery compared with those undergoing open surgery.

Authority is important in medicine. Scientists or clinicians who speak with authority command attention. A paper published in the medical literature must quote in approved form the relevant authorities, and referees will usually be asked specifically to decide whether the author has included the relevant recent references. Each referee is likely to be an accepted authority in the field addressed by the paper. Higher degrees are awarded for distinguished contributions to medical science, and assessment will be in the hands of authorities in the field. Grants for research are awarded by authorities, using criteria which tend to reward reductionist science. Critics of these processes, for example McNeill,[4] point to their narrowness and their self-perpetuating nature. McNeill wants the grant-giving process, particularly where human research is concerned, placed more in the hands of non-medical people. There is a sense that there is something wrong with the notion of authority in medicine. Illich[5] and Goldman,[6] for instance, have made broad attacks on medicine and its claims to authority.

The problems of authority in medicine

It therefore seems timely to re-examine the problems which the medical reliance on authority may be generating, both in the areas of medical research and clinical medicine (which cannot be separated) and to address three questions about the effects of authority.

1. Is it corrupting, in the sense that it allows dishonesty by providing attested precedents for almost any course of action, whether that action represents 'best practice' or not?
2. Does the influence of authority impede the introduction of new methods into medical practice and limit the originality of research?
3. Is reliance on authority dangerous because it encourages members of the profession to turn inward for their guides to action rather than outward to the needs of patients?

Authority can certainly be invoked to support a wide variety of different practices. In the days when surgery was widely used to deal with peptic ulceration, it was possible to quote authoritative support for partial gastrectomy; vagotomy and gastroenterostomy; vagotomy and pyloroplasty; vagotomy and antrectomy; selective vagotomy and drainage; or highly selective vagotomy — each as the 'best' procedure for uncomplicated duodenal ulcer resistant to medical treatment. The problem is that judgments of this kind depend very much on the meaning of the word 'best' in the social context and in the context of individual patients. Best might mean 'associated with the lowest recurrence rate', 'carrying the lowest chance of serious dumping symptoms', 'associated with less malnutrition than other operations' or 'the operation with the lowest mortality'. Faced with these difficult choices, surgeons appealed to the authority of other surgeons who had investigated in a 'scientific' way the effects, the advantages and disadvantages of each operation. Each surgeon chose a 'usual' operation to perform for the 'usual' patient, but varied this choice according to the co-morbidity, the sex, age and weight of the individual patient. This use of authority and the obvious element of preference and choice might seem to support Feyerabend's[7] extreme relativism, which holds that there are no enduring scientific methods or facts, but only perceptions of truth that change with changing times — but it does not. Surgeons do not pick an operation out of the hat when they are asked to intervene in a problem resistant to other means. They use an operation made familiar to them by their teachers and within their surgical scope. They choose that operation from the alternatives because they have heard or read its justification at the hands of an authority. This is in no sense a corrupt process. Any idea that preference based on deference to authority conflicts with a concept of 'best practice' is based on a misunderstanding about the nature of 'best practice'.

There is commonly no single method of treatment which is definitely better than all others when measured by cost–benefit or cost–utility techniques. It is already clear that laparoscopic cholecystectomy is 'better' than the conventional open technique in the early post-operative phase, because patients may return to work within days rather than weeks, and their post-operative pain is demonstrably less. A year later, there are few differences in satisfaction or post-cholecystectomy symptoms,[8] and there is no reason to think that reflux of bile into the stomach and of stomach contents into the oesophagus — both recognised complications of conventional cholecystectomy — will be less frequent in the long term. The serious complication of bile duct damage seems to be more common with the laparoscopic technique. It may well be that the laparoscopic technique will prove to be 'best practice', but the decision to define it in that way will take more time and more evidence than is available at present. Issues of this kind are less easy to resolve than the public may think, but the difficulties lie in the matters themselves, rather than in the attitudes of doctors.

Does established authority inhibit innovation in medicine? There is no denying that track record is used as a criterion for funding research, and in one sense this means that well-established and productive programs continue to be funded at the expense of fledgling or tentative programs. Equally, there is no point in denying the possibility that potentially productive innovations may at times be passed over by granting bodies with limited funds. The film *Lorenzo's Oil* vividly portrayed a medical profession closed to ideas from 'outsiders', and determined that nothing worthwhile could come from people without a specifically medical training. It is easy enough to see how this view arises, but it is based on a misconception. Apart from the specifically human aspects of the sciences of anatomy, pathology and physiology, most medical science has, in fact, been imported from outside medicine. Chemistry, biochemistry, genetics, molecular biology, physics and statistics were not conceived purely for the use of medicine, but without them pharmacology, modern anaesthesiology, synthetic antibiotics, biosynthesised hormones like insulin, endoscopes, prosthetic joints and intensive care units would not exist. Similarly, the clinical trial — the ultimate standard of clinical investigation — would not stand on its present base without the help of statisticians, who began by considering the laws of chance as they relate to gambling and the distributions of characteristics such as chest circumference within populations and expanded their analytical methods into areas such as agricultural yields. The eclecticism of modern medicine is beyond doubt.

There is a specific charge levelled against those with authority within the medical profession: that they dismiss too lightly the claims of alternative medicine. Those who make this charge point out that herbalists, naturopaths, homoeopaths, osteo-paths, acupuncturists, iridologists and others have been in prac-tice for centuries, and that they have a significant body of satisfied clientele. Few medical practitioners deny this, and the move toward 'holistic' medicine reflects the recognition that there is more to healing than the reductionist views of cure, remission or palliation. What really matters in this argument is the medical requirement for evidence.

Medical statistics and the controlled trial have been im-mensely powerful in countering ideology, misplaced commit-ment and pseudo-science. Before Louis made his celebrated examination of the effects of therapeutic blood-letting, it was widely 'known' by both doctors and lay people that blood-letting was a vital part of therapy for most diseases. The influential François Joseph Victor Broussais (1772–1838) taught that all disease is inflammation, for which the remedy must be 'de-pletion' by letting blood. This belief was backed by Broussais' authority, but it was disproved by using statistical methods to test Broussais' claims.[9]

That type of evidential requirement remains one of the essen-tial characteristics of orthodox scientific medicine, and there is no reason why it should not be maintained. If it is seen as a demarcation between medicine and alternative medicine, that is no bad thing. There seems to be no reason why the public should not have a choice between therapies. The rationales, achieve-ments and shortcomings of conventional medicine are measured and available for scrutiny. Therapies of a traditional kind have the support of time, belief in a non-scientific system and another kind of received authority, but their evidential support is usually hearsay and anecdotal. The shortcomings of orthodox medicine are known because they are systematically sought and published. The benefits of alternative methods are 'known' because it is not considered necessary to provide scientific support. It is at this point that the scientific and research attitudes can be seen to provide their most significant input into the discipline of medicine. The requirements that orthodox medicine incorporate more traditional medicine, while not using patients as guinea-pigs to test unproven remedies, are incompatible.

The charge that medicine turns inwards to its own sources of research, and not outward to its constituent population, is perhaps the most serious of all, and the hardest to refute. Toombs documented in detail the failure to communicate between physician and patient because the scientific 'gaze' of the physician does not match the patient's experience of illness.[10] Little[11] examined the breakdown of the humanitarian ethic in medicine, and a number of doctors, as we saw in chapter 1, have written about their own experiences of the inadequacy of medical insight into their own illnesses. It is easy to blame the 'authorities' — the medical faculties for inadequate teaching, the professional bodies such as the learned colleges for failing to insist on proof of communication skills before certification, and professionals individually for becoming dehumanised. The problem is unfortunately much more complex.

The biopositivist model and the hermeneutic tradition

What is at stake is the medical profession's investment in the biopositivist model. Since the days of Claude Bernard, medicine has been seen increasingly in realist, materialist and reductionist terms,[12] and the scientific component of medicine has steadily grown at the expense of the hermeneutic component from which medicine presumably originated. This has been an immensely productive process, and has more than any other single factor contributed to the genuine advances of medicine. Before the first tentative moves toward experimental medicine by such men as Harvey in the 17th century, medicine had made few major advances. For a variety of reasons — religious prohibitions, lack of instruments, theory containment by ancient authority — observations were largely limited to the description of symptoms and signs, and were interpreted using theories that could not be conclusively tested. The advent of critical methods and the evolution of schools of physiology and pathology put the epistemological foundation of medicine on a new base.[9] It is essential to understand the evolutionary significance of this change. The traditional practice involved careful observations of the few vital signs such as pulse and respiration, lumps, tenderness, heat and cold, available to unaided senses; the formulation of diagnosis and prognosis; and the administration of the few treatments whose effects could be observed without instrumental aid (bleeding, incising, excising, purging, deadening consciousness). The success of modern medicine depends almost entirely on its scientific base. The elucidation of causes, the understanding of normal structure and function and of the interrelationships of physiological systems have provided the springs of progress. The dramatic advances in treatment (the technical side of medicine) depend entirely on the epistemological revolution in medicine which has followed the adoption of an ethos of science and technology.

To abandon the biopositivist model would be foolish, but its success has led to the communication difficulty perceived by patients and an increasing number of doctors. Kuhn[13] remarked that 'Although it has become customary, and is surely proper, to deplore the widening gulf that separates the professional scientist from his colleagues in other fields, too little attention is paid to the essential relationships between that gulf and the mechanisms intrinsic to scientific advance.' In Kuhn's view, transition of a pre-science to a science is marked by the appearance and the widening of this gulf, and this is increasingly true of medical science. Success with reductionism and objectivism has emphasised the primacy of the British empiricist philosophical tradition within medicine. The Mannheim and Frankfurt traditions of German philosophy, however, have continued to develop the hermeneutic direction initiated by Heidegger.[12] Gadamer, in particular, has evolved a theory of communication based on 'horizons of understanding'.[14] Habermas has extended this concept by using 'ideology' as a central concept in analysing the processes of communication.[15] Ideologies are sets of beliefs and theories that societal groups use to communicate among themselves and to cement existing power relationships. The meaning of fundamental terms will be coloured by conflicting ideologies. The word 'healing' has different connotations when used by a conventional medical practitioner envisaging a process within the bio-positivist model, and by an advocate of alternative medicine with a 'holistic' concept in mind. Habermas[15] stressed the importance of ideology critique as a basis for human understanding and communication. The relevance for medicine, when it now faces so much informed criticism of its failure to communicate, is very clear.[12]

Faculties of medicine are coming to grips with this problem, but slowly and with incomplete conviction. Harvard University has introduced a major humanistic component to its new pathway. Mayo Clinic has a Socratically conducted ethics and humanities course. At Columbia University Dr Charon's course in understanding the patients' view has achieved a place in the curriculum.[16] The University of Sydney is restructuring its medical course to allow access for those with a graduate degree in the humanities, and plans to stress communication skills in a new graduate medical course. It remains to be seen whether these moves will improve the communication skills of medical graduates or change the orientation of medical research away from its present reductionist objective toward outcome investigations which relate more directly to societal needs, or whether established authority will preserve the *status quo*. There are specific areas of difficulty which confound even fluent and skilled communicators, and which need to be learned. It is hard to break bad news, hard to deal with hostility and uncertainty, and very hard to communicate information that is probabilistic. There is very little in conventional medical courses that would equip graduates to be comfortable with information that expresses uncertainty. In the next chapter, we will examine specifically the problems of explaining outcomes that have only a probability of occurrence, to patients who want certainty.

NOTES

1. Kitcher P. Authority, deference, and the role of individual reason. In: McMullin E, ed. The social dimensions of science. Notre Dame, Indiana: University of Notre Dame Press, 1992:244–71.
2. Gieryn TF. The ballad of Pons and Fleischmann. In: McMullin E, ed. The social dimensions of science. Notre Dame, Indiana: University of Notre Dame Press, 1992:218–43.
3. Lakatos I. Falsification and the methodology of scientific research programmes. In: Lakatos I , Musgrave A, eds. Criticism and the growth of knowledge. Cambridge: Cambridge University Press, 1974:91–196.
4. McNeill PM. The ethics and politics of human experimentation. Cambridge: Cambridge University Press, 1993.
5. Illich I. Limits to medicine: medical nemesis, the expropriation of health. Calder & Boyars, 1976.
6. Goldman L. When doctors disagree: controversies in medicine. London: Hamish Hamilton, 1973.
7. Feyerabend PK. Against method. London: New Left Books, 1975.
8. Wilson RG, Macintyre IMC. Symptomatic outcome after laparoscopic cholecystectomy. British Journal of Surgery 1993; 80:439–41.
9. Canguilhem G. Ideology and rationality in the history of the life sciences, Goldhammer A, trans. Cambridge, Massachusetts: MIT Press, 1988:41–50.
10. Toombs SK. The meaning of illness. A phenomenological account of the different perspectives of physician and patient. Dordrecht: Kluwer Academic Publishers, 1992.
11. Little JM. Medicine and the humanities — the nature of the nexus. Mayo Clinic Proceedings 1993; 68:921–4.

12. Wulff H, Pedersen SA, Rosenberg R. Philosophy of medicine, 2nd edn. Oxford: Blackwell Scientific Publications, 1990.
13. Kuhn TS. The structure of scientific revolutions, 2nd edn. Chicago, Illinois: University of Chicago Press, 1970.
14. Gadamer H-G. Truth and method, 2nd edn. Glen-Doepel W, trans. London: Sheed & Ward, 1979.
15. Habermas J. Knowledge and human interests, Shapiro JJ, trans. London: Heinemann, 1972.
16. Charon R. Doctor–patient/reader–writer: learning to find the text. Soundings 1989; 72:137–52.

5

Probability: Master or Servant?

Explanation is a complex matter, and the source of much philosophical dispute. Some philosophers of science have claimed that only deductive–nomological explanations (by inference from a law of nature and a statement of initial conditions) have real validity, and that all apparently different types of explanation have deductive roots. More generally, however, other types of explanation are recognised. These include the probabilistic or statistical, causal, genetic and teleological (the theory that anything can be understood only by considering the ends it is aiming at). The importance of probabilistic explanation in medicine demands attention.

The status of probability within epistemology has been a matter of debate among the philosophers of science.[1] Some have followed Keynes in defining probability as a logical relationship between propositions. They would say that a proposition has a certain probability by virtue of its relationship to a set of propositions that constitute a covering law. Thus, if two parents carry a recessive gene for a genetically determined disease, the children have a 0.25 probability of suffering that disease, because the Mendelian laws of genetic inheritance provide a model which infers that result. Others, following Venn, advocate a frequency theory of probability, claiming that all probability statements imply that a class of events occurs within another class of events with a frequency that expresses a probability of occurrence. The cure rate for Dukes Stage C carcinoma of the colon is about 30%, and this figure is reached by observing the course of as many appropriate patients as possible, rather than by reference to an underlying mathematical law. Probabilism in either form as an epistemological theory has been strongly criticised by many philosophers, among them Popper[2,3] and Foley,[4] while Hempel[5] has argued for the epistemic contribution of probabilistic inference.

Medical graduates think of probability most strongly in terms of statistical probability, and believe that studies which produce statistically significant differences prove that one treatment is better than another, with an appropriate degree of confidence. The familiar statement along the lines that 'Treatment A produced more rapid resolution of disease X than treatment B ($p < 0.05$)' convinces many that the case is now closed, and that treatment A must now be preferred to treatment B, regardless of what was thought before the current trial. The matter is less straightforward in reality.

Frequential and subjective probability

It is necessary to distinguish between two different concepts of probability, both of which are important to the theory and practice of medicine.[6] The first can be called frequential probability. It describes the frequency with which an event is likely to occur in a long run of trials. Both the genetic events and the percentage of cancer survivors mentioned above are examples of frequential probability. The second is subjective probability. This describes the degree of certainty with which a person believes a hypothesis to be true. In clinical diagnosis, for example, finding an elevated alpha foetoprotein above 200 IU/mL in a person with chronic active hepatitis B who also has a mass in the liver on a CT scan might make clinicians 95% sure that the liver mass is a hepatocellular carcinoma. In order to determine this level of confidence with any accuracy, we would have to test the degree of commitment by a manoeuvre such as a standard gamble.[7] In this procedure, a person is offered different odds against winning a gamble, until a point of indifference is reached — that is, the chance of winning ceases to outweigh the cost of the gamble. Foley[4] criticised probabilism of this kind for its lack of consistency within the belief systems of an individual, but clinicians have to rely on feelings of relative certainty in many of their daily decisions.

The empirical tradition — the concept that objective evidence outweighs subjective feelings and intuitive responses — is very strong in medicine. Scientifically oriented modern clinicians prefer to know that 30% of patients having liver resection for isolated metastases from colonic cancer will survive five years, rather than have a general impression that patients who undergo liver resection are better off than those who do not, under similar clinical conditions. Survival statistics, success rates for treatment, the accuracy of diagnostic tests and population norms are all expressed as frequential probabilities, based on empirical observations of more or less large populations. Rationalists in medicine also produce frequential probabilities when they predict, using models, what the limiting frequency of occurrence of a disease should be. The predicted reduction of mortality from cholesterol-lowering programs expresses this kind of deduced frequential probability based on an underlying theory and a mathematical model. Eddy[8] considered this kind of data as the salvation of medicine that now costs too much to continue without control. Precise frequential knowledge of success rates, he claimed, can be continually updated by computers using Bayesian or other similar programs to assimilate new information.

Objective frequential probability, however, does not translate smoothly to subjective probability, and it is subjective probability that clinicians use in practice. The medical consultation does not involve large groups of people. It concerns a person

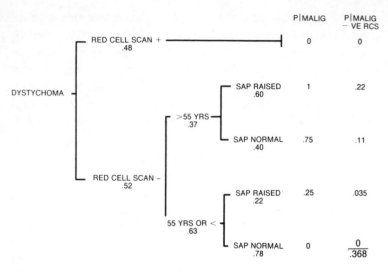

	P|MALIG	P|MALIG − VE RCS
RED CELL SCAN + .48	0	0
SAP RAISED .60	1	.22
SAP NORMAL .40	.75	.11
SAP RAISED .22	.25	.035
SAP NORMAL .78	0	0 .368

Figure 5.1 Diagnosis using a decision tree. A dystychoma is a solid lesion in the liver found by chance on organ imaging. 'Red cell scan +' refers to a positive red cell scan, which indicates the diagnosis of hepatic haemangioma. 'Red cell scan −' refers to a negative red cell scan which indicates that there is some pathology other than haemangioma. '>55 yrs' and '<55 yrs' refer to patient age at the time of presentation. 'SAP' is serum alkaline phosphatase, a liver enzyme which can be easily and cheaply estimated. The figures beneath each heading refer to the probability of each characteristic in the whole population, while the right-hand column (labelled 'P\|MALIG') gives the risk of malignancy associated with the chain of characteristics to the left. Thus, 52% of individuals presenting with the problem of an unexpected solid lesion in the liver will have a negative red cell scan. Of this 52%, 37% will be aged more than 55 years. Of those over 55 years with negative red cell scans, 40% will have a normal SAP. 75% of those with negative red cell scans over the age of 55 years and with a normal SAP will have a malignant tumour.

who is 'ill' or who may become ill, a clinician, and the relationship between the two.[9] Clinicians 'know', for example, that 17% of all patients with the chance finding of an asymptomatic liver mass on CT or ultrasound will suffer from a malignancy of the liver, either primary or secondary. They know that those patients who are over the age of 55 have a much higher probability of malignancy, and that nearly all patients older than 55 who have an elevated serum alkaline phosphatase will have malignancy.[10] They also know that patients with positive red cell scans all have haemangiomas, and that none of these are malignant. Thus they start with a subjective probability of 17% for a malignant diagnosis, based on their knowledge of the prior frequential probability, and modify their belief in that diagnosis as more diagnostic information becomes available. A trigger point may be reached in the protocol of investigation, when clinicians feel entirely confident that a diagnosis has been reached. The red cell scan, for example, may be positive, and clinicians may reassure their patients that no further tests need be done, and that the condition is entirely harmless. This process is shown as a decision tree (Figure 5.1).

All too often, however, clinicians work under a veil of ignorance, faced with a number of possible diagnoses and with no time to investigate and refine diagnosis. They may have to act without clear direction from their own subjective probabilities for each diagnosis because the penalties for inaction in the face of each possible diagnosis are too great. A young, immunosuppressed person dying in an intensive care unit from adult respiratory distress syndrome may be suffering from overwhelming septicaemia, endotoxaemia or cytomegalovirus infection, among many other possibilities. Such a patient will receive multiple modes of treatment because death will soon follow unless the triggering cause can be reversed.

Probability and practice

These examples illustrate the difference between frequential and subjective probability in clinical medicine. Communicating the nature of these probabilities is very difficult. In confronting a person with operable secondary liver cancer, clinicians cannot simply advise that the 'best' treatment will certainly be a liver resection. At best, they can express their conviction that the patient will benefit from surgery as being equivalent to a conviction that they will draw a red marble from a bag containing 70 black marbles and 30 red ones. The clinicians' level of conviction that this is the best advice to give will depend on many factors, such as their appreciation that the only five-year survivors have undergone resection, and that those in whom the procedure fails are no worse off than if they had no surgery (a debatable premise — the post-operative recovery consumes a significant part of the time left to the patient). Clinicians may try to stage the disease more accurately, and to allocate the patient to a subgroup of those with liver metastases. They may note that there are five separate areas of secondary tumour on the CT scan, and that only about 5% or fewer with more than three secondaries live five years.[11] Confronted by a single patient, however, clinicians cannot rely on frequency of occurrence in many trials. The patient is unique, and clinicians can advise solely on the basis of their own subjective assessment of the probability of benefit. Further, the clinicians' reading of the odds and the weight they assign to benefits may not match the patient's subjective assessment of risks and weights. People differ in their risk-taking behaviour. Goodin,[12] in analysing the use of heroic measures in medicine, stressed that 'people have trouble assimilating and acting rationally upon propositions about low probability events ... The dramatic being more memorable than the mundane, people tend to overestimate the probability of the former events relative to that of the latter.' As Hollis[13] said: 'Medicine has more to it than applying decision theory to diseases.' There is no 'best practice' that will suit every patient and every doctor.

This does not deny that there is an obligation on the medical profession to accumulate better frequential statistics about disease incidence and prevalence, the accuracy of diagnostic tests and the outcomes of treatment of diseases. The decision-making theorists in medicine have made real contributions to the understanding of the medical process and the mix of reasoning and intuition that is expressed in medical judgment.[14] The advent of

cheap and powerful computers has stimulated interest in computer-aided diagnosis and decision-making, and many of the
programs that have been developed use Bayes' theorem to update diagnostic and therapeutic information in the light of new
information from clinical studies. Interested readers are referred
to Dawson-Saunders and Trapp[15] for a useful introduction to
this field.

Very briefly, Bayes' theorem deals with the modification of
probability that occurs as evidence becomes available. Thus, a
clinician might reason that the (prior) probability that a new
patient suffers from hydatid disease before anything else is
known about that patient may be 1 in 100 000. If the patient has
a relevant history of exposure to dogs on a sheep station in
childhood, the probability may increase to 1 in 500. If the sheep
station was in an area where the disease is known to be common
among sheep, the probability may become 1 in 100. If the
patient has pain in the right upper quadrant of the abdomen and
the physical finding of an enlarged liver, the chances might be 1
in 10. If the patient brings an ultrasound examination showing a
cyst in the liver with daughter cysts within it, then the (posterior) probability would be more than 95 in 100.

Bayes' theorem allows the more precise quantification of
these probabilities. More importantly, it provides a mathematical illustration of the reasoning that clinicians use in their daily
problem-solving. Information derived from Bayes' theorem (or
from any of the other methods for deriving the same posterior
probabilities from the prior probabilities) can be summarised in
the form of a decision tree. Figure 5.1 shows an example, setting
out the probabilities derived from empirical studies of patients
with solid lesions in the liver discovered by chance during investigations for unrelated symptoms. Algorithms of this type help
clinicians to construct protocols that will lead most effectively
and efficiently to a definitive diagnosis. They also provide frequential probabilities from which to derive a degree of confidence in the subjective probabilities assigned by clinician and
patient. Specialists in nuclear medicine, for example, commonly

report the results of perfusion/inhalation lung scans by stating the frequential probability of association between a particular scan appearance and the presence of a pulmonary embolism. That frequential probability needs to be translated into a subjective probability in the context of other clinical features, such as age, presence of malignancy, post-operative state, prior venous disease. When clinicians judge that a critical level has been reached in their own perception of subjective probability, they may decide to treat the patient with heparin. Therefore it is the subjective probability of a diagnosis that guides action, even though the objective studies on which clinical confidence is built produce frequential data.

The probability of a hypothesis

There is a further, and very important, aspect of probability in medicine. That is the subjective probability that is assigned to the truth of the hypotheses upon which clinicians base their decisions in every activity of medicine. Like all biological systems, humanity is irretrievably stochastic, and we are very far from having a deterministic or genetic explanation of every disease. The very scale of the human genome project — a massive and expensive international collaboration between scientists attempting to map the entire human genetic structure — suggests that it will be a very long time before scientists unravel the geography and interactions of genes. In the meantime, clinicians will have to continue to use probabilistic data, and to hold to the 'working' hypotheses in clinical medicine with variable conviction. Modern medicine is firmly convinced that the biopositivist model, with its empiricist, reductionist and determinist base, is the one to follow. Clinical trials are the scientific paradigms in clinical medicine. Clinical scientists report their results with p-values attached, and p-values cause immense and subtle confusion.

The p-value, as it is commonly used, records the frequential probability of generating such a result under the null hypothesis in a large series of similar trials if they could in fact be carried out. *P*-values do not represent the level of confidence that we should feel in the truth of the hypothesis under examination.[6] That level of confidence — the subjective probability — largely depends on the medical theories and models in which clinicians believe. The result of a 'good' trial by a recognised authority may make clinicians modify their level of subjective probability of the truth of a hypothesis, as Levi[16] pointed out, but this underlying 'credal commitment' is likely to be established by prior adoption of a system of beliefs about the way the body functions in health and disease, and about the reasonable and effective methods that can legitimately be used to influence bodily function. Modifications to credal commitment follow a process akin to the Bayesian one, and some philosophers believe that it is possible to quantify these changes using classical Bayesian algorithms.

An example may help. Let us suppose that a clinician reports at a meeting that a local application of common salt in hypertonic solution cures cancer of the skin. He has information on 25 patients with basal cell cancer, 18 of whom have 'done very well' without progression of disease for five years. Of 25 basal cell cancers in other patients managed by observation alone, none has stabilised in this way, and all have shown increase in size. The result is statistically significant, with $p < .001$ on Fisher testing. This does not mean that the listeners should adopt the conclusion that common salt controls skin cancer with more than 99% certainty. The result simply shows that fewer than 1 in 1000 similarly conducted studies will produce a similar result by chance. But if the treatment method does not fit any underlying theory that most doctors would accept, there must be healthy scepticism about the result. The most logical response to such a report would be a determination to repeat the study under more stringent conditions. Just as happened with the Pons and Fleischmann report on cold fusion, when scientists see a claim that is far from all that is accepted about a field of study and practice they see it as either very wrong or extremely important.[17] Lakatos[18] pointed to the importance in research programs of the 'negative heuristic', the central tenets which must not be challenged, since they determine the direction and success of the program. These are usually the hypotheses assigned the highest subjective probability. Even very low p-values in single studies may not change the levels of credal commitment; the evidence has to be very strong, as the credibility of a successful program may be at stake.

Explaining probabilities

These complexities of probability make communication between doctors and patients even more difficult than they already are. Clinicians are armed with frequential probabilities as their 'objective' data, but are forced to rely on subjective probabilities when they deal with one patient. They cannot try their treatment 100 times on each patient. They must therefore express their level of confidence in each choice, or offer the patient an array of data and ask that the patient choose the treatment. In other words, clinicians either dissociate themselves completely from the procedure of choosing (which is impossible, and is certainly not what the patient wants from a professional whose help is sought), or act under some degree of paternalism, however mild and however much solicited. The presentation of the facts and the selection of the facts to be presented must depend to some extent on individual clinicians and their commitment to one hypothesis over another. Given the same facts — survival after radical resection for liver cancer, or quality of life after amputation, for example — three clinicians may give differing advice because they differ in their views about life-worth-living, sanctity of life and conflicts between what they perceive as patient needs and wants. It is inevitable that patients are confused by the probabilistic nature of the 'scientific' data presented by doctors, and become increasingly confused if they seek multiple opinions. To seek an opinion that offers realistic hope in understandable terms is a natural ambition for any person with a serious illness. When probabilistic science appears to produce opinions that seem pessimistic and indefinite, it is hardly surprising that patients turn away from orthodox to alternative medicine. In Thurber's book *The Thirteen Clocks*,[19] the princess is unable to start the clocks by touching them. The answer (according to the logic of a character called the Golux) therefore must be *not* to touch them, and indeed they start when she holds her hand just far enough away from each clock: 'Now let me see,' the Golux said, 'If you can touch the clocks and never start them, then you can start the clocks and never touch them. That's logic, as I know and use it.' Goluxian logic often underlies the appeal to alternative medicine. Those who know orthodox medicine cannot cure; therefore those who do not know must have the cure. One breakdown in communication leads to another. The illogic of this logic needs to be understood with sympathy, not dismissed with incomprehension and contempt.

Decision theory and the Bayesian approach to probabilistic data may be helpful in some situations, but no amount of figuring will persuade all patients that they are receiving the 'best' and the most empathic advice. In particular, persuading a distressed patient, in pain and faced, for example, with the possibility of losing a leg, to help in the decision-making process by examining the situation with the standard gamble is scarcely likely to help resolve the profoundly emotional situation. To produce a solution based on such concepts as quality-adjusted-life-years may be helpful to those who need to look at the macro and microeconomics of medicine.[20,21] But the solution may not be helpful when the figures suggest something which runs strongly against intuition. At a meeting on decision theory, I took part in an exercise which examined amputation of the leg for diabetic small vessel disease. The analysis by the lecturer was immaculate in its formal structure, but it reached a result diametrically opposed to my own solution, because the lecturer used a value for his assessment of quality of life after amputation which was quite unlike the one that I developed after years of work with amputees. I do not know what the 'right' answer was, but it seems unlikely that the patient would know either. Further, an adjustment of the values assigned to quality of life after treatment may make a radical difference to the final decision, despite suggestions to the contrary by Lockwood.[20]

Unsatisfactory as it may be, probability permeates the whole of clinical medicine and most of biological science. It is certainly true that more data are needed about the outcomes of disease, both treated and untreated. But there is also a sense in which the increasing subtlety of classifications — while it defines more sharply subgroups with better or worse prognosis — adds to the difficulties of understanding and communication. Understanding the reasons for these difficulties is the first step towards overcoming them. Medical education needs to address the problems generated by the clinicians' need to explain their explanations. There are those who feel that these problems may be solved by more and better data, and that there are mathematical ways to express medical information which will lead to better explanation and better understanding of what it is that medicine achieves. In the next chapter, we will examine these claims in more detail.

NOTES

1. Passmore J. A hundred years of philosophy, 2nd edn. Harmondsworth: Penguin, 1968:412–23.
2. Popper KR. Conjectures and refutations: the growth of scientific knowledge. London and New York: Routledge, 1989:285–92.
3. Popper KR. Objective knowledge: an evolutionary approach. Oxford: Clarendon Press, 1979:141.
4. Foley R. Probabilism. In: French PA, Uehling TE Jr, Wettstein HK, eds. Midwest studies in philosophy vol xv: the philosophy of the human sciences. Notre Dame, Indiana: University of Notre Dame Press, 1990:114–29.
5. Hempel CG. Philosophy of natural science. Englewood Cliffs, New Jersey: Prentice-Hall, 1966:47–69.
6. Wulff HR, Pedersen SA, Rosenberg R. Philosophy of medicine — an introduction, 2nd edn. Oxford: Blackwell Scientific Publications, 1990:172–202.

7. Clarke JR. A scientific approach to surgical reasoning. V. Patients' attitudes. Theoretical Surgery 1991; 6:166–76.
8. Eddy DM. Medicine, money and mathematics. American College of Surgeons Bulletin 1992; 77:36–49.
9. Little JM. The problem of the clinical process — a Popperean analysis. Theoretical Surgery 1993; 8:146–50.
10. Little JM, Kenny J, Hollands MJ. Hepatic incidentalomas: a modern problem. World Journal of Surgery 1990; 14:448–51.
11. Little JM, Hollands M. Hepatic resection for colorectal metastases — selection of cases and determinants of success. Australian and New Zealand Journal of Surgery 1987; 57:355–9.
12. Goodin RE. Heroic measures and false hopes. In: Bell JM, Mendus S, eds. Philosophy and medical welfare. Cambridge: Cambridge University Press, 1988:17–32.
13. Hollis M. A death of one's own. In: Bell JM, Mendus S, eds. Philosophy and medical welfare. Cambridge: Cambridge University Press, 1988:1–16.
14. Lorenz W. Current status of theoretical surgery: marginal example or model for systematic medical decision-making? Theoretical Surgery 1992; 7:135–6.
15. Dawson-Saunders B, Trapp RG. Basic and clinical biostatistics. London: Prentice-Hall International, 1990:229–63.
16. Levi I. Direct inference. Journal of Philosophy 1977; 74:5–29.
17. Gieryn TF. The ballad of Pons and Fleischmann: experiment and narrative in the (un)making of cold fusion. In: McMillin E, ed. The social dimensions of science. Notre Dame, Indiana: University of Notre Dame Press, 1992:217–43.
18. Lakatos I. In: Lakatos I, Musgrave A, eds. Criticism and the growth of knowledge. Cambridge: Cambridge University Press, 1974:91–196.
19. Thurber J. The thirteen clocks. Harmondsworth: Penguin 1962.
20. Lockwood M. Quality of life and resource allocation. In: Bell JM, Mendus S, eds. Philosophy and medical welfare. Cambridge: Cambridge University Press, 1988:33–56.
21. Broom J. Good, fairness and QALY's. In: Bell JM, Mendus S, eds. Philosophy and medical welfare. Cambridge: Cambridge University Press, 1988:57–74.

6

Autonomy and a Calculus of Clinical Benefit

There is a justifiable major interest in defining and measuring medical outcomes.[1] It is not really possible to apply standard econometric techniques to the medical process when there are no measures of benefit or harm that result from the process. Traditionally, clinicians have expressed their results in terms of mortalities, survivals over standard times and complication rates. More recently, researchers have tried to express outcomes in less familiar ways — as utilities or as measures of quality of life. Unfortunately, these measures are difficult to use. If they are kept simple, they are too crude to detect small differences. The refined measures are so complex that they will find support only with research workers with particular studies in mind.

Quality of life

Quality of life was discussed briefly in chapter 5. Although the concept is controversial, there is at least some agreement on an operational definition. Quality of life is considered to consist of three domains — the psychological, the social and the physical. Many measures have been proposed for each domain. For example, physical well-being can be assessed by mobility and the activities of daily living; the psychological domain by anxiety, mood and cognitive performance; and social integration by the degree of support needed and provided and by the level of social interactions. A fourth domain is usually added for the specific symptoms that dominate individual disease states. For example, dysphagia and pain need particular consideration when clinicians consider the palliative treatment of carcinoma of the oesophagus, whether they address the problems of one individual or study the results of treating many.

Many scales have been developed. Some are for specific purposes (for example, the Priestman and Baum scale for cancer patients)[2] and others for more general application (for example, the Quality of Life Index of Spitzer and his co-workers).[3] Interested readers are referred to the review by Wood-Dauphinée and Troidl[4] and to the review by Bullinger.[5] More recently, the importance of time has been recognised, and the Quality-Adjusted-Life-Year[6] and the Time-Quality-of-Life unit[7] have been developed to incorporate this additional parameter into quality of life measurement. While all these measures have been used enthusiastically by some workers, they have not become part of standard clinical research. It is clear that measures of quality of life, despite intensive developmental work, still leave major questions unanswered. In particular, a patient's attitudes to his or her particular future, to the impact of altered function and to the altered feelings that accompany disability are not well measured by current scales.[8] There remains doubt and disagreement about the attributes to be included and how they should be scored. There persists an intuitive doubt that the complexity of the subject will always be too great for anything other than academic clinical research, and that quantification of quality may not be conceptually possible.

Autonomy

There may also be an advantage in considering autonomy as an additional measure to quality of life. I am not using the word 'autonomy' in the Kantian sense, which denies any supreme moral authority beyond the individual conscience. I am using it in the more legal or political sense of at least partial self-government for the individual, meaning the capacity to make any informed decision, any potential choice within the bounds of human capacity and the bounds of social constraint. It is certainly not deontological autonomy, but has some of the characteristics of relativist autonomy and some of social autonomy.[9] ('Deontology' is the ethical view that duty is the basis of morality.) It is the autonomy described by Dworkin[10] when he wrote: 'The central idea that underlies the concept of autonomy is indicated by the etymology of the term: autos (self) and nomos (rule or law) . . . There is a natural extension to persons as being autonomous when their decisions and actions are their own.' Dworkin also said something of fundamental importance: 'Liberty, power and privacy are not equivalent to autonomy but they may be necessary conditions for individuals to develop their own aims and interests, and to make their values effective in the living of their lives.' Unquestionably, 'complete' autonomy is not attainable. We cannot all climb Mount Everest, although the decision to make the attempt is theoretically available to all people who are physically and mentally fit enough. Murder, theft and dangerous driving, on the other hand, are unsociable acts and are not available for reasonable free choice. This is the paradox of freedom, and has been dealt with at length and frequently by other writers.[11]

Autonomy, in practical terms, might be defined as the freedom to make realistic choices against a background of good physical and mental health and an awareness of the well-being that accompanies good health. It is the potential to do anything that a human being can do, and an awareness that this potential exists for that individual. Autonomy in this sense will be restricted by physical and mental defects and by intercurrent illness. It can also be restricted by medical treatment, and herein lies its potential sensitivity to the benefits and defects of the medical process. Not only could the advantage or disadvantage of treatment be gauged by measures of autonomy before and after treatment, but the adverse impacts of investigation and surveillance could also be measured in the same way.

Illness limits total autonomy.[12] Even a common cold or an ingrown toenail will limit individual choices that a person can make, because of the sore throat or the painful foot. This does not say that illness automatically makes all independent choices unavailable. Someone who is the victim of intolerable suffering may make an autonomous choice to commit suicide, but such a decision is mandated by a loss of options and by a significant reduction in total autonomy. There is a distinction between the total, ideal autonomy of the healthy person, which includes an autonomy of physical action, and the autonomy of choice that may remain for the severely ill and the disabled. The recent case of a woman in Canada who expressed a desire to end a life made unacceptable by amyotrophic lateral sclerosis is one of many examples of the distinction between autonomy of choice and autonomy of physical action.

We must also observe a distinction between independence and autonomy. Autonomy reflects the potential to choose. Independence reflects the ability to survive (and perhaps flourish) without additional physical, emotional or financial help from an outside agent. It is possible for someone to be independent in the activities of daily living, but not to be autonomous, because of a requirement for regular medication or other medical review and intervention. Consider, for example, the cases of an amputee, a patient with liver metastases and a regional perfusion pump implanted beneath the abdominal skin, and a patient with symptomatic hypertension controlled by beta blockers. Each may lead an 'independent' life of good quality at home, caring for themselves and continuing to earn a living. But each has forfeited some fraction of total autonomy. Each may be 'benefiting' from treatment in terms of past symptoms and future life expectancy and quality, but each has paid a price in the currency of autonomy. None of them can sever their relations with the medical profession without risking some aspect of their health and well-being. For each, quality of life may be excellent, but autonomy is limited. Quality of life indices measure something which differs from indices of autonomy. Combining measures of both may well provide a fuller picture of illness and its treatment.

It is also possible to use the concept of autonomy to measure and explain costs and benefits. Take the example of a patient with symptomatic angina and left main coronary artery disease with a single demonstrable narrowing. Conventional wisdom says that such a patient has a good prognosis with or without surgery, and that the only reason for intervention would be a failure of medical therapy.[13] Individual patients, however, may see the choice quite differently if autonomy becomes part of the discussion. At the cost of some weeks of diminished autonomy, surgery may free the patient from the long-term loss of autonomy required by the needs for continued medication, repeated visits to a doctor and the requirement for available medical care while travelling, all of which reinforce the 'sick role'.

This last issue raises the question of informed consent, a topic which will be examined in more detail in chapter 9. There have been criticisms of the validity of a concept of patient autonomy in the medical relationship, because there is a limit to the understanding of medical issues in the lay mind.[8] Given the profound complexity of the information to be handled in most major medical decisions, consent can at best be no more than partly informed. Thus, the patient's autonomy of choice is not complete, since the elements of the choice remain partly obscure. Paradoxically, the introduction of the concept of autonomy into the medical discussion may increase patient autonomy by defining benefits and disadvantages more clearly. Furthermore, a measure of degree of autonomy could be useful as an end-point for clinical trials involving many patients, and might distinguish subgroups of patients with equivalent quality of life scores who have in fact benefited more than others.

I do not propose to suggest a detailed methodology that might lead to an 'autonomy index', and I do not have the skills to do so. A much oversimplified approach suggests that such an index might examine the impact of illness, treatment and medical surveillance on the scope of choice in the domains of daily domestic routine, daily occupation, recreation and special events such as holidays and travel. Clinicians or research workers could then ask themselves such questions as 'How far will this treatment go toward restoring autonomy?' or 'How much will this surveillance regime interfere with autonomy for any benefit achieved?' Such an approach has been suggested by Toombs.[8] Regimes could be compared on these bases, and ideal managements defined by their capacity to restore full autonomy. It seems likely that few medical interventions will measure up to that standard, and this appreciation could be important in conceptualising the role of medicine in health and sickness. It would be constructive to identify and eliminate regimes — such as the routine screening with carcinoembryonic antigen levels of patients after resection of colorectal cancer[14] — that reduce autonomy while producing no demonstrable benefit.

The possibility of a clinical calculus

Hayek,[15] as we saw in chapter 3, dismissed as 'scientism' attempts to employ the scientific method to examine social issues, regarding such exercises as misleading and as having no validity. Hayek believed the scientific method is legitimately available only for examining the relationships between external physical objects and their phenomena. The relationships between people (sociology, psychology) and between people and objects (economics, environmental studies) are not suitable for objective study and the formulation of laws that have the epistemological validity associated with the physical sciences. This view of the scientific method has been attacked by Tiles[16] and Harré,[17] among others.

Hayek's view may be right in a formal sense, but it does nothing to solve the pragmatic problem faced by those who try to bring formalism and science, however imperfect, into clinical medicine. The central problem for clinical scientists is the need to make decisions from moment to moment based on probabilistic and incomplete knowledge. For this reason alone, clinical medicine has to give inferences more authority than they may deserve. To complicate the epistemological issue, many medical decisions are value-laden, and depend to a varying extent on the society in which the practitioner works. For example, Western societies have a view of the breast which is different from that of Chinese societies, and breast conservation in cancer management is viewed differently by the two cultures. In the West, women commonly seek breast reconstruction after breast removal. In Chinese communities, breast loss is not seen as the end of femininity, and reconstruction is seldom sought. The problem of defining 'best practice' is consequently difficult, and may be impossible without reference to each individual patient.

There is little question that Western medicine needs a way to examine its achievements and shortcomings. Each country is convinced that the health bill is too high, and each talks of 'rationing' or 'rationalisation', of cost containment, efficiency, cost-benefit, best practice and so on. The dubious sciences of economics and managerialism are brought to bear on the dubious science of medicine. Despite isolated instances of success in government intervention (the Oregon scheme seems to be partially successful),[18] it is hard to see any movements within medicine or health which appeal to both patients and practitioners. The progress of technology and the dissemination of high level skills create an expectation in both clinicians and patients that anything is possible and that everything should be available. The truth is that Western societies can no longer afford to support these expectations.

Some degree of market regulation seems to be almost inevitable. It is doubtful that a government in the Western world could survive complete deregulation of all health services. Even a free market would still need information about the achievements and expectations of medical practice if it was to become and remain profitable. In other words, even private entrepreneurs would need to know what was 'effective' in medical treatment and what was not. Whoever runs medicine will need the same information — what can be achieved, and how much it will cost.

Surprisingly, remarkably little is known about what can be achieved, and there is no close agreement on a method by which to calculate the costs. The outcomes of medical treatment have been measured in various ways, many of which are of doubtful relevance, while costs are difficult to measure because of the enormous indirect costs of research, development and technology use that underpin the apparently simple delivery of a given medical service.

Survival and intermediate outcomes

To recapitulate material from chapter 1, survival has been used for many years as the measure of 'success' of a medical intervention. Sophisticated analytical methods are available[19] to compare survival data which may distinguish one treatment as the 'best'. Actuaries have used expectation of life as one measure of the health of a community, and we know that the mean expectation of life at birth has increased by about 26 years during the 20th century in a Westernised community.[20] This very real achievement is probably reaching a level of diminishing returns, and its impact can only be appreciated in retrospect, when the data is available for analysis. Because data on length of life are characteristically probabilistic and long-term, clinical researchers have tended to use intermediate effects[21] as endpoints rather than wait for the true effects on quantity and quality of life. This concentration on intermediate effects reflects the culture encouraged by the grant-giving process, which assesses merit partly by the feasibility of obtaining a result from the investigation within a 'reasonable' time. But how can we express outcomes in a way that is comprehensible? Do they even allow quantification, or can we only 'understand' them?

Benthamism: quantifying the unquantifiable?

Utilitarianism has been remarkably durable, despite the strong criticisms of its ethical assumptions and potential consequences. Bentham was taken to task by his contemporaries for his obsession with lists and classifications, and for his attempts to quantify qualitative experience. Dinwiddy[22] wrote that 'many people . . . have regarded Bentham as the source of much that is soulless and materialistic in modern culture'. Nevertheless, his attempts to quantify individual pleasure and pain in terms of intensity, duration, propinquity (of future pain or pleasure) and certainty of achievement need to be taken seriously. Measures of these dimensions were multiplied to produce an index of pleasure or pain, and multiplied by a further measure of extent when a community of individuals would be affected by a decision. Bentham[23] himself recognised that intensity would be difficult to measure because of the variation between people, but also insisted that, however imperfect the measures, there was value in 'the application . . . of arithmetic to questions of utility'. He said: 'at any rate, in every rational and candid eye, unspeakable would be the advantage it will have over every form of argumentation in which every idea is afloat, no degree of precision being ever attained because none is ever so much as aimed at'.

Bentham's difficulty with intensity has been answered to some extent in the context of clinical medicine by the development of quality of life scales which assign a numerical value to a qualitative data set. There does not seem to have been any work so far seeking to quantify autonomy, but that should not deter an attempt to develop the general principles of a clinical calculus.

A clinical calculus

A calculus for assessing choices between medical treatments would need to include:
1. positive measures of:
   a. expectation of real benefit;

b. prolongation of life;

c. improved quality of life;

d. significant protection against disease or complications;

2. negative measures of impact of treatment on:

   a. quality of life;

   b. autonomy;

   c. cost;

3. a measure of extent, e.g. incidence or prevalence.

Since all of these measures could be seen as reflecting some such concept as utiles,[24] they could be considered in a single calculus (in Benthamite terms). Thus, the factors for an individual in the calculus would include the following.

1. A disease D, with untreated life expectancy L under depreciated quality of life Q and depreciated autonomy level A, and with risk R of developing serious complications that would further shorten life or depreciate quality of life and level of autonomy. Utile value for the untreated state would then be expressed as $L(Q+A)(1-R)$, since quality of life and autonomy could be considered as at least partly independent: it is possible to imagine a reasonable quality of life with diminished autonomy, and *vice versa*.

2. Treatment T of duration X, with probability P_1 of achieving life expectancy L_t, probability P_2 of quality of life Q_t, probability P_3 after treatment of autonomy level A_t, risk of serious and enduring complications R_t, at depreciated costs C_{t1} during treatment and C_{t2} long-term. Long-term utile value could then be calculated from:

$$P_1 . L_t(P_2 . Q_t + P_3 . A_t)(1-R_t)$$

From this must be subtracted the negative impact of the acute phase of treatment, where X is the duration of treatment, Q_{at} is quality of life during treatment, and A_{at} is the level of autonomy during treatment. This quantity then becomes:

$$-X[(Q-Q_{at})+(A-A_{at})]$$

if the baselines for calculation are taken as the levels of quality of life and autonomy at the start of treatment.
3. Calculation of marginal cost–benefit ratio requires division of this quotient by the sum of a measure of cost for both acute and continuing treatment.

The assessment formula for any given treatment T can then be expressed as a utile–cost ratio:

marginal utile(T)–cost ratio =

$$\frac{[P_1.L_t(P_2.Q_t+P_3.A_t)(1-R_t)-X\left\{(Q-Q_{at})+(A-A_{at})\right\}-L(Q+A)(1-R)]}{(C_{t1}+C_{t2})}$$

where utile(T) represents the marginal utility value of treatment T. In other words, the denominator in this equation (marginal utile(T)) represents the marginal utility of treatment minus the negative utility of the morbidity of treatment, and minus the utility of the natural history of the disease. It is stressed that this algorithm represents a *marginal* utility, which will reflect gains achieved by treatment over the natural history of the disease.

This algorithm expresses a utility–cost ratio (that is, utiles per unit cost), rather than the more familiar cost–benefit ratio. This utile–cost ratio expresses the utility per health dollar spent on each individual. Multiplication of this ratio by a measure of incidence or prevalence would provide an index of utility for the community over a period of time. Total cost could be estimated from $F(C_{t1}+C_{t2})$, where F is an appropriate measure of frequency.

Is a clinical calculus practicable?

The algorithms suggested in this chapter are relatively simple, although they may make assumptions that are of debatable validity. Will it really be possible to generate a reproducible autonomy index? Is it possible to consider that a treatment produces a quality of life identifiable by a single score? Surely the quality of life changes with time and at times as complications develop or remissions occur. The correct way to depreciate the value of life years is not yet agreed. Attempts to deal with this problem of non-uniformity over periods of time have been made by the concept of the QALY[25] and the time-quality-of-life unit.[7] Again, the mathematics on which these concepts are based is simple. There are also other (perhaps even simpler) ways of examining material of this kind, particularly using decision trees.[26] It is not algorithms that stand in the way of numerical analysis of qualitative issues.

Despite the self-evident economic and social chaos affecting clinical medicine and the political sensitivity of distribution and funding of health, there is remarkably little commitment by physicians and surgeons to developing a science of outcomes and outcome economics. Even if the algorithms are shown to be of limited use for describing something that clinicians, funders, administrators and patients can understand, the exercise of developing them is useful in alerting everyone to the components of the medical transaction and its costs. Generating the kind of data that could be handled in even these simple ways will take time and the ingenuity of intelligent people. The issues are large ones — economics, equity and the whole epistemology of clinical science. Research in these fields lacks the glamour of molecular biology, but it is just as important. The difficulty of the research is no reason to avoid it. Clinical medicine ought to be judged by its outcomes, and granting organisations ought to encourage a scientific culture in which outcome research has proper priority. It is also important to understand that the examination of outcomes, particularly bad ones, may have other benefits.[27]

For the moment, doctors must recognise that clinical trials, decision-making techniques and algorithms that take note of autonomy and quality of life can still only generate probabilistic information. This is one of the major problems for clinicians and patients. It is easy enough for clinicians to present their patients with a set of probabilities that are as accurate as possible. No amount of accuracy will compensate for the insecurity of probabilities. Probabilities are confusing to patients, as well as threatening. Modes of communicating probabilities have been researched by those interested in decision-making. The standard gamble[28] and the time trade-off[29] are two techniques that have been proposed, but neither is easy enough to understand or to implement to be of practical use in daily clinical encounters. Add to this the need to discuss outcomes in terms of poorly defined measures of quality of life or utilities as well as probabilities, and the confusion is made infinitely worse. Nor is the confusion eliminated by the best probabilistic data that can be generated. It is the need to discuss uncertainties in terms of unmeasured qualities, all of central importance to patients, that causes the confusion, resentment and anger that so often beset clinical encounters, particularly when a serious illness is at issue. Better data may help, but will not solve the problem until all uncertainty can be eliminated.

Better data and better mathematics, therefore, cannot solve communication problems. What else might help to regulate and direct the transactions between doctors and patients? The doctor–patient relationship is influenced by professional ethics at every level. The ethical movement has indeed had a profound effect on the practice of medicine and medical research. The next two chapters will examine some of the ways in which modern medicine has been changed by the rise of the ethical movement, and the potential of ethics to solve some of the problems that arise in the medical relationship.

NOTES

1. Much of the text of this chapter first appeared in Little JM. The potential contribution of autonomy to a calculus of clinical benefit. Theoretical Surgery 1994; 8:221–6. It is reproduced here by kind permission of the editors of that journal.
2. Priestman TJ, Baum M. Evaluation of quality of life in patients receiving treatment for advanced breast cancer. Lancet 1976; 2:899–901.

3. Spitzer WO, Dobson AJ, Hall J, et al. Measuring the quality of life of cancer patients. A concise QL-index for use by physicians. Journal of Chronic Disease 1981; 34:585–97.

4. Wood-Dauphinée S, Troidl H. Endpoints for clinical studies: conventional and innovative variables. In: Troidl H, Spitzer WO, McPeek B, et al, eds. Principles and practice of research: strategies for surgical investigators. New York: Springer-Verlag, 1991:151–68.

5. Bullinger M. Quality of life: definition, conceptualization and implications — a methodologist's view. Theoretical Surgery 1991; 6:143–8.

6. Loomes G, Mackenzie L. The use of QALYs in health care decision making. Social Science and Medicine 1989; 28:299–308.

7. Little JM. A method of calculating the value of palliative care of cancer patients. Australian and New Zealand Journal of Surgery 1987; 57:393–7.

8. Toombs SK. The meaning of illness. A phenomenological account of the different perspectives of physician and patient. Dordrecht: Kluwer Academic Publishers, 1992.

9. Jensen UJ, Mooney G. Changing values: autonomy and paternalism in medicine and health care. In: Jensen UJ, Mooney G, eds. Changing values in medical and health care decision making. John Wiley & Sons, 1990:1–15.

10. Dworkin G. The theory and practice of autonomy. Cambridge: Cambridge University Press, 1988:108.

11. Popper KR. The open society and its enemies, vols I & II. Princeton, New Jersey: Princeton University Press, 1971.

12. Cassell EJ. The nature of suffering and the goals of medicine. Oxford: Oxford University Press, 1991:27.

13. Pentecost BL. Myocardial infarction. In: Wetherall DJ, Ledingham JGG, Warrell DA eds. Oxford textbook of medicine, 2nd edn. Oxford: Oxford University Press, 1984, 13:174–87.

14. Bruinvels D, Stiggelbout AM, Kievit J, van Houwelingen JC, van de Velde CJH. Follow-up of colorectal cancer patients: a meta-analysis. Poster presented at Fourth Biennial Conference, European Society for Medical Decision Making. Marburg, FRG, 14–16 June 1992.

15. Hayek FA. The counter-revolution of science: studies on the abuse of reason. Indianapolis: Liberty Press, 1979.

16. Tiles M. Method and the authority of science. In: Phillips Griffiths A, ed. Key themes in philosophy. Cambridge: Cambridge University Press, 1989:31–51.

17. Harré R. Realism, reference and theory. In: Phillips Griffiths A, ed.

Key themes in philosophy. Cambridge: Cambridge University Press, 1989:53–68.

18. Haas M, Hall J. The Oregon plan. New South Wales Public Health Bulletin 1992; 3:50–1.

19. Armitage P, Berry G. Survival analysis. In: Statistical methods in medical research, 2nd edn. Oxford: Blackwell Scientific Publications, 1988:421–39.

20. Fries JF. Aging, natural death and the compression of morbidity. New England Journal of Medicine 1980; 303:130–5.

21. Eddy DM. Medicine, money and mathematics. American College of Surgeons Bulletin 1992; 77:36–49.

22. Dinwiddy J. Bentham. Oxford: Oxford University Press, 1989.

23. Bentham J. Works of Jeremy Bentham, Bowring J, ed. Edinburgh, 4:542.

24. Edwards W. Theory of decision making: a general review. In: Edwards W, Tversky A, eds. Decision making. Harmondsworth: Penguin, 1967:29.

25. Allen D, Lee RH, Lowson K. The use of QALYS in health service planning. International Journal of Health Planning and Management 1989; 4:261–73.

26. Fox HC, Blatt MA, Higgins MC, Marton KI, eds. Medical decision making. Boston: Butterworths, 1988.

27. Little JM. Decisions in clinical management: a case scenario. Medical Journal of Australia 1993; 158:204–7.

28. In this context, the standard gamble provides a method of assessing the subject's feelings about the outcome of decisions which involve certainty in one direction (death from liver cancer within two years), and uncertainty in another (a 25% chance of living five years with surgery, a 2% chance of dying from the surgery). The odds are varied in the decision arm with uncertain outcome until the subject can no longer perceive any benefit from choosing either of the two options. These probability levels are then used to estimate the utility that a decision to operate might have for the subject.

29. Time trade-off estimates the utility of methods of treatment in chronic illness by presenting the subject with a list of options which express the amount of time that a patient would be prepared to trade off his or her total length of life for a given period of good quality life. Again, this result can be used as a measure of the utility of a proposed treatment which may, for example, produce early benefit with risks of later disability.

7

Ethics and the Definition of Professionalism

The word 'profession' can mean many things. Here it is being used in the sense of the OED definition of 1541: 'A vocation in which a professed knowledge of some department of learning is used in its application to the affairs of others, or in the practice of an art founded upon it'.[1] In this context it was first applied to divinity, medicine and the law. This chapter will preserve the earlier meaning, and neglect the current habit of using the word 'professional' to mean 'paid' for doing something, in contrast to the sense of 'amateur' or 'dilettante'. There are many other occupations, however, which also involve academic training, and equip graduates to make a living by employing a corpus of knowledge in the service of others who do not have the education or the time to master this knowledge. Computer programmers, systems analysts, accountants, airline pilots and paramedics are all knowledge workers (in the sense used by Drucker[2]), and it is difficult to see a valid distinction between the old learned professions and the new owners of useful knowledge. It still seems worthwhile, however, to examine the basic concepts of professionalism, and to accept that there are some vocations that can be understood only by appreciating their dependence on a knowledge paradigm, a commonality of purpose, an ideal of service to others and an ethical under-pinning to practice.

Herbert Spencer in 1936 traced the history of the professions, and pointed out that they were at one time considered to be those occupations that were compatible with a gentlemanly life, involving neither manual work nor direct commerce.[3] Thus, physicians could practise a profession at a time when surgeons could only practise a trade, and internal medicine was placed on a collegial basis far earlier than surgery. Adam Smith[4] insisted that people's need to place their health and welfare in pro-fessional hands meant that professionals could not be 'people of a very mean or low condition'. Furthermore, 'Their reward must be such . . . as may give them that rank in society which so important a trust requires.' This meant that professionals should not have to compete in the market place, but should be well compensated for their irreplaceable services. Times change, and the social standing of learned professionals has declined, while that of business people has improved. While professionals still have generally good standing, the incomes that they earn can be well below those of their commercial contemporaries, whose purchasing power and financial importance now set the social trends. In addition, most professionals work hard and usually do have to compete to secure larger practices and enough money.

The learned professions have, therefore, to find something else by which to define themselves, and most recently have con-centrated on the part of the above definition which specifies their application of learning to the affairs of others. This idea of service is central to the way that medicine, for example, would lay claim to a special status within the community. The service ideal focuses on the welfare of the recipients (the patients) rather than the corporation (the medical profession), and it defines minimal standards of education and competency by ensuring that the learned colleges certify that these standards have been met before clinicians start unsupervised consulting practice.

Because an ideal of service is embedded in the thinking of the learned professions generally, their codes of ethics have particular importance. These codes are often tacit and paradigmatic, but they signal the underlying sense of morality which the influential members of the profession consider necessary to regulate the practice of their members. While there is a wide spectrum of ethical theories and practices, the behavioural ethical codes of the professions generally stress moderation in self-advertisement, moderation of fees, respect for the autonomy of clients, respect for other members of the profession, confidentiality and an abhorrence of fraud. In addition to certifying the competence and ethical awareness of those trained within the profession, the collegial bodies provide protection against invasion by the unqualified, thus guaranteeing a benign restriction of trade in the interests of standards.

Ethics and the definition of professionalism

Ethics thus constitute a significant part of the definition of what it is to be a professional. The accepted ethical matrix (whether enunciated or tacit) declares the presence of a relationship of trust, a declaration which is different from the guarantee available to buyers in commercial transactions. Commercial customers can inspect before they buy. There are commercial guarantees and legal codes to protect buyers. Lawyers, however, cannot guarantee to win cases, nor doctors to cure a condition without complications. The contract between professionals and clients is one of trust. It is assumed that lawyers or doctors will guarantee to do their best, and to apply their knowledge and experience to the case in hand — but they cannot guarantee the outcome. Nor is their product standardised. Individualism in the professions still matters.[5] Those who can choose want the 'best' barrister or the 'best' surgeon because they recognise that some individuals achieve better results than others. It is this individualism, and the high value put on it by the public, that makes ideals like uniform 'best practice' so difficult to achieve. And even if 'best practice' is successfully introduced as a pattern of medical behaviour, individual performance in the human and hermeneutic aspects of medicine will continue to distinguish between one clinician and the next.

In commercial transactions, the ignorance of consumers may raise various difficulties. A couple buying their first house, car or computer could be persuaded by an unscrupulous salesperson to spend more than they can afford, or they may be persuaded to buy defective goods which they do not know how to recognise. The doctrine of *caveat emptor*, however, is no longer so easily accepted, and consumer rights and consumer organisations now provide some protection against commercial dishonesty. Furthermore, potential purchasers are commonly advised to seek expert help from building inspectors and motoring organisations when they propose to buy houses and cars. Commercial contracts can be standardised, and the products in a commercial transaction can be scrutinised by experienced buyers or their agents. These opportunities for objective assessment are less readily available for professional transactions. Reputation, qualifications, training history, professional history and publications may all help to identify an expert worthy of consultation, but given the individuality of practitioners and clients, there is no way to know whether the outcome will satisfy a client before the surgery is done or the case is heard in court. There are some matters that draw legal sanctions, for example malpractice, incompetence and fraud. But the skill of professionals and their capacity to fulfil the needs of clients simply have to be taken on trust, and it is this implication of the transaction that professional ethics tries to safeguard. However much professionals may respect the autonomy of their clients, they are always asked to assume some degree of solicited paternalism when their opinion is sought. The clients are asking the professionals to act as de facto extensions of the clients' intelligence, skills and knowledge into an area of relative ignorance. Even if advice is rejected, questioners surrender a small part of their autonomy by asking a professional opinion, and this surrender is made necessary by a relative ignorance and by a comparative incapacity in the matter at hand. Within the client–professional relationship, the needs of the client are paramount. The definition of those needs and the capacity to meet them will vary from society to society, and from time to time. A doctor can advise a patient that a symptomless cancer of the breast detected on screening needs to be removed, because the doctor can foresee the symptoms it will cause and the shortening of life that will result. The patient's decision on whether to agree to treatment depends partly on the trust she feels in the person giving that advice. If professionals seriously breach that trust, they will evoke the sanction of their collegial group, as well as the sanctions of the law. Thus, a doctor guilty of scientific fraud or a lawyer who has misappropriated funds may both lose their registration to practise medicine or the law because, it is reasoned, neither can be trusted implicitly to observe the ethically imperative constraints and demands of professional practice.

Collegiality or conspiracy?

While the regulatory activities of a professional body may protect the public, there are negative aspects of collegiality. The ethics of client management represent a profession's recognition of its social obligations; the ethics of intraprofessional relationships are also important. Respect of health care workers for each other is a part of this ethic within medicine. Sometimes it seems that this ethic of respect and support overrides the obligations of respect and support for clients and the community. The Chelmsford Hospital episode in Australia (see chapter 1) apparently uncovered a system of collusive support for practitioners within the mainstream who were practising an aberrant medicine, and harming their patients. Once these activities were brought into the open, the regulatory activities of the collegial bodies moved into action and various punishments were devised, both legal and professional. But we can ask why the self-regulatory activities were so slow.

The answer lies less in an ethic of mutual protection at all costs than in the tacit assumption that highly qualified and experienced professionals are bound to observe the ethics of their profession. As rumours about malfeasance begin to circulate, they are met with the frank disbelief of fellow professionals. It is hard to accept that standards of ethical behaviour which have been defined since the days of the ancient Greeks can be disregarded so irresponsibly. Once the evidence reaches a critical mass, however, the professional bodies react (sometimes quite punitively — as shown by the recent deregistration of an eminent senior Australian doctor for scientific fraud — see chapters 1 and 3) to restore trust. By then it is often too late, and the public has good grounds to accuse the professions of active or passive collusion in protecting their members. The mechanisms of self-regulation have not yet been perfected, largely because they must be created where ethical commitments conflict with one another. The same comment can be applied to child abuse or violence within marriages. Friends and neighbours are often incredulous when they find that they have been mingling with someone who seems monstrous beneath the cold and highly filtered lights of the law and the media.

Ethics and the balance of welfare

The ethics of professional behaviour are determined by the need to balance the power of the professional against the needs of the client. In this particular context, the payment system has been seen as a problem. In the 1930s, Laski took an extreme ideological view when he wrote: 'They [the professionals] cannot give of their best to the civilisation in which they play so large a part so long as their members offer their services for private hire or sale.'[6] Few would now agree with this opinion, but payment for professional service does pose conceptual problems, since a fee for service will generally increase according to the complexity of the service, and total income increases with the number of services performed. Both these considerations might encourage overservicing. The professional bodies, therefore, have to strike a balance between the free market and market regulation, insofar as they can influence the fee structure of their members at all. The professional bodies have no legal power to enforce moderation, and depend on the tacit agreement of their members to accept standards of ethical behaviour which help to maintain the reputation of the profession. The professional bodies have to work by consensus. They have no absolute moral authority.[7] They do not, and could not, insist on altruism to the exclusion of income, nor do they discourage the competitive development of private practice. What they try to encourage is the preservation of the service ideal, which must be seen in the context of the purpose of the profession. In medicine, the purpose is the improvement, maintenance or restoration of individual health. Clinicians try to achieve this by treating individuals; public health officers aim to improve individual health by improving the health of the community. The energies of a disparate group of people are directed by this common purpose, whatever their motives may be for practising medicine. Uniformity of practice is an ideal which is unlikely to be achieved because of the diverse beliefs and commitments of practitioners and patients, but uniformity of purpose can be assumed — and this purpose does not depend on the method of payment for the services provided.

Ethics and the ethical movement

There seems, therefore, to be a paradox. The identity of the professions is much bound up with appropriate ethical systems, yet the collegial bodies have no moral authority and limited legal powers. They depend for their good name on the collaboration of their members, and it is surprising that there are so few aberrations in the practices of the thousands of professionals with variable commitment to and understanding of the ethical principles involved. In medicine, the ethical movement has developed remarkably in recent years, and it seems worthwhile to examine the nature of current ethical thinking and its application to medicine.[8-11] To do this, we will need to describe further some of the underlying principles of ethical thought (which owe much to Kant[12]), since confusion of ethical principles leads to the endless confusion of argument from different premises.

Ethics is that branch of philosophy which examines the nature of the 'good'. It is synonymous with moral philosophy. It distinguishes between decisions and acts that are good in themselves and those that are good as a means. Penicillin is good as a means of treating pneumococcal pneumonia in an 80-year-old stroke victim who can no longer care for herself or communicate with family and friends, but the decision not to treat such a person may be seen by ethicists and family alike as good in itself.

The word 'ought' also occupies a central place in ethical thinking. Ethicists are much concerned with the logical status of ethical laws and with the forces of obligation that encourage people in a society to follow these laws. Ethical laws do not necessarily have legal sanction, nor do they have the empirical backing which endorse laws of nature. The nature of the imperative which encourages men and women to behave in moral ways remains a problem for philosophers and ethical thinkers within professions like medicine. Kant distinguished the categorical from the hypothetical imperative,[12] and his thinking has influenced ethical writing ever since. Doctors confronted with an elderly stroke patient with pneumonia may reason that, for moral reasons, life must be saved at all costs, and that they must therefore give penicillin. In doing this, they are bound by what they believe to be a categorical imperative. If, however, they give penicillin because they fear that the family may charge them with neglect if they fail to treat the patient, they are acting under the constraints of a hypothetical imperative — one which depends on a consequence which may or may not follow. Confronted with a choice of this kind, clinicians' actions may be determined as much by the law and the attitudes of the society in which they work as by the moral dimensions of the problem.

The origins of morality are difficult to categorise.[13,14]

1. Intuitive responses are important, although philosophers have rejected intuitionism as the sole basis of moral thought. Most people, for example, feel that physical and mental cruelty are intrinsically bad, and that there is a categorical imperative to abstain from and condemn cruel acts.
2. Religions have been and still are powerful moral forces. In the West, the Judaeo-Christian legacy still determines many aspects of moral thinking and judgment, despite a decline in formal religious observance.
3. Emotivists take a view that is influenced by logical positivism. They say there are no methods of empirical confirmation for ethical hypotheses, so there is no point in discussion. Although this stance is no longer common among philosophers, the scientific and empirical nature of modern medicine has probably contributed to the slowness with which ethical thinking has permeated medical thinking.
4. Ethical naturalists claim that there is no difference between empirical facts and value judgments. They claim that evaluative words like 'good', 'bad' and 'ought' can be expressed in utilitarian terms such as 'happiness' and 'quality of life' to increase the empirical content of ethical discussion.

Ethics as a branch of philosophy exists at three levels at least.

1. Descriptive ethics, like any empirical endeavour, simply documents, classifies and counts ethical issues.
2. Meta-ethics is a branch of philosophy which examines the logical status and the meaning of ethical statements and their underlying concepts.
3. Normative ethics examines the basis for the formulation of moral principles, seeking justifications for the way that

people and societies actually formulate moral codes and view moral behaviour.

Normative ethicists tend to espouse either utilitarian or deontological ethics. Utilitarians stress the outcomes that follow moral choices: how much good, or harm or happiness. Deontologists say that qualities such as justice, honesty or respect for autonomy are categorical imperatives, regardless of the outcomes. A strict deontologist might argue, for instance, that patients must be told the truth about their health, even if telling will distress patients and their families. Truth, in this view, overrides any desire to avoid anguish. Both utilitarian and deontological thinking attempts to provide a rational basis for values that are intuitively judged to be 'right'.

Deontological or utilitarian attitudes can be further classified as individual, egoistic or universal according to the scope of their effects. They can be further considered by their relevance to a particular act or to a general rule. Doctors who decide to withhold treatment from a particular elderly stroke patient with pneumonia on the grounds that this particular patient no longer has a life worth living, and that the family have said that they will be glad to see the patient's suffering ended, are making an individual act utilitarian decision. They may not generalise their decision to conclude that every elderly stroke patient should be excluded from treatment for pneumonia: the decision is to apply to this single act of withholding treatment. It is utilitarian because it considers the consequences in terms of human suffering and happiness. Doctors who hold that it is intrinsically and always wrong to carry out abortion adopt a universal rule deontological stance, while one who waits until morning to operate on a patient with appendicitis may be following egoistic act utilitarian principles. Such classifications are often imprecise, but awareness of these differing bases for moral thought can be helpful in understanding why differences in values may prove irreconcilable when protagonists argue from different premises.

Kant insisted on the deontological basis of ethics, rejecting the consequentialist views of utilitarianism, which were elaborated in the 19th century by Bentham[15] and J.S. Mill.[16] The concepts of autonomy and free will were also fundamental to Kant's view of morality. Humanity comprises individuals with the capacity for choice. Ethics are constructed as a social reality, because the rightness of certain actions and the wrongness of others are appreciated *a priori* and intuitively. Modern medical ethics also put great store on respect for autonomy.

While Kant stressed individuals and their contribution to the justice of society, Rawls[17] took justice as his starting-point: 'Justice is the first virtue of social institutions, as truth is of systems of thought.' His deontological view of morality led him to suggest a social contract, under which people have equal rights and as much liberty as the rights of others will allow. Society is to be organised to maximise the benefits to those least advantaged, and contributions to social welfare and advancement are to be rewarded.

Daniels[18] suggested that an ethical system should recognise the validity of moral intuitions, and find a place for them in the scheme of practical ethics. An ethical system should be coherent and based on a set of moral principles, be they utilitarian or deontological, and on acceptable background theories about humanity and society — like those of Rawls. Social contract theory implies that medical professionals should place more emphasis on justice and respect for individual autonomy than on strictly utilitarian judgments. Other theories insist that ethical systems should be based on fundamental human rights.

Practical ethics and medicine

It seems necessary to examine these fundamentals of ethics, because the subject is complex and important. In the daily practice of medicine and medical research, the background theory is rarely examined in any detail, even by those who are involved in advising their colleagues about the ethical basis of practice. It is not surprising that professionals should seek practical guidelines for action, rather than discussions of competing theories — discussions that are never resolved. In medicine, the result has been a 'cookbook' approach, with the definition of a few key issues that should be considered when any ethical decision must be made. Four leading maxims are commonly cited as the cornerstones of medical ethical thinking and behaviour.[11]

1. All medical decisions and actions should be guided by the intention to do good and not harm — the principles of beneficence and non-maleficence.
2. Respect for autonomy is paramount. Unsolicited paternalism is not justified. Solicited paternalism — when patients hand decisions to clinicians — can be seen as an expression of the autonomous patients' right to choose. True paternalism — in the case of incompetent patients — is also justified, although its boundaries are ill defined and there are legitimate questions about the meaning of incompetence. This issue is further examined in chapter 8.
3. Practitioners, involved in a tacit social contract, must provide their services with justice to all, regardless of social, financial, racial, religious or other potential prejudices. The distribution of services must also be regulated with justice — a requirement that is particularly difficult to manage. Even in countries with comprehensive health systems, the wealthy live significantly longer than the poor.
4. All practitioners should act always with professional competence, since that is what patients expect, and that is what the collegial system within medicine purports to provide. Professional competence includes efficiency in dispensing service with the least waste of time and money.

Granted that there is some agreement on these four principles, how can ethics be brought into professional practice effectively? The history of the ethical movement in medicine illustrates some of the problems in maintaining an ethical hold over professional activity.

The *stele* of Hammurabi from about 2000 BC prescribes rewards and punishments for effective and ineffective treatment, but it does not touch matters that we might regard as ethical. The Hippocratic Oath (probably cast in its present form in about 360 BC, well after the death of Hippocrates) deals briefly with doctor–patient relationships, the types of treatment doctors will not undertake, the need for confidentiality and discretion and the obligations of the collegial structure of the profession. The Hippocratic injunctions against abortion and the absolute prohibition against shortening life have retained some of their categorical imperative to this day. The Oath remained the central ethical document in medicine until the mid 20th century, although medical practitioners never formally took the Oath. Surgical texts of the Middle Ages concentrated mainly on social bearing and avoiding trouble, offering detailed advice on illnesses that doctors should refuse to treat, lest they lose their reputation by undertaking treatment and failing to cure. Louis XIV's surgeon thought it reasonable to practise on condemned prisoners before operating on the king's anal fistula. Harvey needed no ethical approval for his animal experiments. The English Royal College of Physicians was founded in 1518 and the Royal College of Surgeons in the late 18th century, but their first concerns were with standards rather than with other ethical matters, and they concentrated on training and licensing.

The modern ethical movement in medicine began with the Nuremberg trials after the Second World War.[10,11] The knowledge of what had happened in the medical 'experiments' of concentration camp doctors so horrified the public and the medical profession that the Nuremberg Code was promulgated in 1947 to govern research involving human subjects. The Code stressed that subjects should be fully informed of the purpose and risks of the investigation proposed and should give consent of their own free will; that researchers should ensure that there were no undue risks involved; and that any risks should be clearly outweighed by potential benefit.

Despite the publication and wide dissemination of the Nuremberg Code, some investigations in the 1950s and 1960s failed to observe the guidelines. The best known is the Willowbrook trial, set up in 1957, in which a group of mentally retarded children in New York State were deliberately infected with hepatitis virus so researchers could study the course of the disease. The research workers argued that most children would contract the disease anyway, and that the experimental group would be better cared for than in the general wards. Ethicists and other medical researchers objected that informed consent could not be obtained because of incompetence; that parents giving consent on their children's behalf were subject to unfair coercion because they feared that their children would not be well treated in the general wards; and that an experiment of this kind did nothing to solve the hygienic failures responsible for the spread of hepatitis in the general wards. The Tuskegee study, which ran from 1932 to 1972 in the southern United States, is less well known, but raised at least as many ethical problems.[19] Four hundred black men with syphilis were left untreated so that the natural history of the infection could be documented by physician–scientists of the US Public Health Service. The subjects were not told that treatment was being withheld. They had regular examinations and blood tests. Penicillin became available during the study, but was not administered to those in the study.

In 1965, the World Medical Association issued the first version of the Helsinki Declaration, prescribing rules for the conduct of human medical research. The Declaration has been revised several times, most recently in 1989. In 1982, the World Health Organization (WHO) and the Council for the International Organizations of Medical Sciences (CIOMS) issued their *Proposed International Guidelines for Biomedical Research Involving Human Subjects*. CIOMS published *International Guiding Principles for Biomedical Research Involving Animals* in June 1984. Peter Singer has articulated the case for animal rights in his book *Animal Liberation*.[20]

Despite all this interest and despite the many statements of ethical concern, problems continue to surface. In Australasia alone, the Chelmsford Hospital incident involving unproven deep sleep therapy for psychiatric illness (see chapter 1), the Auckland National Women's Hospital longitudinal observation of women with in situ carcinoma of the cervix without their informed consent and the McBride case involving scientific fraud (see chapters 1 and 3) make it very clear that the ethical component in medicine is not given the respect that it deserves, and that the medical profession cannot be complacent about its unwritten ethical standards. There is still a gap between concept and practice.

Is there a future for ethics in the professions?

Most doctors seem willing to accept that autonomy must be respected, and that unsolicited paternalism should be avoided. Most have attended meetings at which ethical issues have been discussed. Informed consent is part of any invasive treatment and any investigative protocol. Ethics committees examine and must approve clinical trials and animal experiments. Review committees check that animal care is of good standard. This openness and these critical processes can only do good, and there seems little doubt that they will continue and increase in their scope. But the expansion of the ethical movement has its problems, and no one should expect Utopian consequences.

In the first place, compulsory ethical review of scientific programs can stifle progress as effectively as withdrawing grants. Ethical values change rapidly, and it is possible for a productive and large animal transplant program to be closed after five years because new standards of animal care have been promulgated. Constraint inhibits scientists, many of whom now spend more than 50% of their time meeting the requirements of the many agencies to whom they are responsible for the conduct of their research. This does not question the importance of ethical standards in research, but it does raise important questions about the main purpose of scientific endeavour and training.

A second, and very important, issue concerns the concept of 'best practice'. There can be no question that obtaining the best possible result in the most efficient way is one of the central ethical tenets of any profession. But the definition of 'best practice', as we have seen, is extraordinarily difficult, and the concept raises questions about who should decide what constitutes the 'best' and the 'most efficient'. Ideally, there should be consensus between those who fund medicine, those who practise medicine and those who receive its services. The Oregon scheme[21,22] (based on a concept of universal provision of medical care to a certain level and the right to purchase higher level services) suggests that consensus can be achieved in small states with an enlightened legislature, but in large and pluralist societies such agreement is hard to win. It is far easier to agree that 'best practice' is desirable than it is to define it.

The third issue, which is closely related to the issue of best practice, returns to the necessity to act with incomplete information when making decisions in medicine. Approximately 34 000 new articles are added to the medical literature each month.[23] New computerised methods of information handling are impressive, but they do not solve the problem of information flood which afflicts most professions. Eddy[24] foresees a society in which there are information systems available on every doctor's desk, systems which will update themselves as new information comes into the literature around the world, and which will offer up-to-the-minute advice about likely diagnoses and the best method of treatment. These systems will be incredibly complex if advice relevant to all communities and all individuals is to be generated, rather than advice that is relevant only within those countries and communities that can afford to develop the appropriate systems. If they are to be really respected, pluralism and individual autonomy will add another and daunting dimension to decision technology.

Much of the uncertainty about best practice in medicine reflects the inadequacy of research into treated and untreated outcomes. The ethical movement in medicine will need to take this problem in hand. Without knowledge of outcomes, doctors remain on uncertain grounds when they advise patients on the most effective treatment for conditions as widely separated as low back pain and metastatic liver cancer. Distributional justice and professional competence cannot be guaranteed unless doctors know what they achieve by one treatment instead of another. Scientific reductionism is powerful and effective in medicine, but there is a need for other types of research if the ethical basis which in some ways defines the profession is to be confirmed and strengthened.

These are technical problems for the ethical movement. Of far greater importance is the absence of the moral authority to ensure that ethical practice is the norm.[7] Pluralism makes secular moral consensus difficult, however much the Oregon experience[21] may reassure us that it can be achieved. But even if a majority consensus can be achieved, the dissenting minority do not have to conform unless there are legislative sanctions, in which case the issue is no longer ethical, but legal. This in turn raises a new set of problems about the governance of professions. At present, there is tension between those who contend that the motives and aims of professionals will ensure progress and a majority adherence to ethical practice, and those who contend that measures of professional output should be used to change and regulate professional structures and activities. The first may be seen as a deontological view of a profession, according to which adherence to a set of categorical imperatives, such as honesty, confidentiality and a determination to act in the best interests of clients, can be expected from a majority of practitioners. This concept assumes that the ultimate aims of the profession are in the interests of the community (regardless of the motivation of individual practitioners), and that the activities of the profession will inevitably be regulated from within as long as the purpose of the profession remains useful to the community it serves. By contrast, a utilitarian view insists that outcomes should be measurable and measured, and that these measures of output must be used to control the profession. The utilitarian view predicates external assessment and control of professions, and inevitably suggests legal sanctions over many aspects of professional activity. The professions clearly prefer the deontological view, and do in fact use mechanisms to maintain the integrity and relevance of what they do. The utilitarians feel that self-regulation is suspect, and there seems little doubt that external interference will increase in the next generation in all professions and in many aspects of professional activity. The professions would do well to emphasise their ethical base and to develop their internal monitoring systems if they are to retain credibility. Unless they do this and can be seen to do it effectively, the law will replace ethics, and the scope of the professions and their standing will be seriously eroded. A bioethics committee has been seen as the way the medical profession can show the sincerity of its attempts to scrutinise the moral difficulties of modern medical research and practice. This claim will be examined in the next chapter.

NOTES

1. Shorter Oxford English Dictionary, Onions CT, revd and ed. Oxford: Clarendon Press, 1933.
2. Drucker PF. The coming of the new organization. Harvard Business Review 1988 January–February: 45–53.
3. Spencer H. The principles of sociology, vol III, part VII. London, 1896.
4. Smith A. An inquiry into the nature and causes of the wealth of nations, vol 1, 5th edn, Cannan A, ed. London: Methuen, 1930:107.
5. Marshall TH. Class, citizenship and social development. New York: Doubleday, 1965:158–79.
6. Laski H. The decline of the professions. Harper's Monthly Magazine, November 1935:656–7.
7. Engelhardt HT Jr. National health care policy: the moral issues. American College of Surgeons Bulletin 1993; 78–4:10–14.
8. Wulff HR, Pedersen SA, Rosenberg R. Philosophy of medicine — an introduction, 2nd edn. Oxford: Blackwell Scientific Publications, 1990:172–202.

9. Glover J. Causing death and saving lives. Harmondsworth: Penguin, 1977.
10. McNeill PM. The ethics and politics of human experimentation. Cambridge: Cambridge University Press, 1993.
11. Campbell A, Gillett G, Jones G. Practical medical ethics. Auckland: Oxford University Press, 1992.
12. Kant I. Fundamental principles of the metaphysics of ethics, 10th edn, Abbott TK, trans. London: Longmans, Green & Co, 1940.
13. Foot P, ed. Theories of ethics. Oxford: Oxford University Press, 1967.
14. Williams B. Ethics and the limits of philosophy. London: Fontana/ Collins, 1985.
15. Dinwiddy J. Bentham. Oxford: Oxford University Press, 1989.
16. Mill JS. On liberty. Quoted in: Warnock M, ed. Utilitarianism. London: Fontana/Collins, 1962:136.
17. Rawls J. A theory of justice. Oxford: Oxford University Press, 1972.
18. Daniels N. Reflective equilibrium and Archimedean points. Canadian Journal of Philosophy 1980; 10:83–103.
19. Katz J. Abuse of human-beings for the sake of science. In: Caplan AL, ed. When medicine went mad: bioethics and the holocaust. Totowa, New Jersey: Humana Press, 1992:233–70.
20. Singer P. Animal liberation. New York: New York Review/Random House, 1975.
21. Thorne JI. Oregon pro: as the nation waits, Oregon moves forward. American College of Surgeons Bulletin 1993; 78–3:8–14.
22. Liu JT-Y. Oregon con: Oregon's experiment: just another Medicaid cutback. American College of Surgeons Bulletin 1993; 78–3:8–14.
23. Arndt KA. Information excess in medicine: overview, relevance to dermatology, and strategies for coping. Archives of Dermatology 1992; 128:1249–56.
24. Eddy DM. Medicine, money and mathematics. American College of Surgeons Bulletin 1992; 77:36–49.

8

The Bioethics Committee

It is, for all practical purposes, impossible to do anything within a profession these days without the blessing of an ethics committee. In medicine, the ethics industry has been particularly penetrative. Any new research project will need ethical review, using guidelines such as those issued in the Helsinki Declaration.[1] Members of the Ethical Review Committee will decide whether the risks of the program will outweigh the potential benefits, whether risks have been reduced to an irreducible minimum, whether patient autonomy has been respected, whether informed consent will be obtained, whether the principles of justice have been respected and whether the criterion of professional competence has been satisfied. They will also decide whether it is actually ethical to run the study, in the light of what is known about present methods of treatment. They may consider whether it would be justified to divert funds from other and proven methods of treatment. They may also consider the ethical problems associated with using experimental animals. They may even criticise the experimental design for faults which would reduce its efficiency and the likelihood of producing a result.

This reflection on ethical issues has been salutary. A repetition of the Willowbrook trial[2] (where intellectually disabled children

were deliberately infected with hepatitis) would be most unlikely in a major hospital in the 1990s, and animal management
has improved enormously as a direct result of the Animal Rights
movement. Institutional requirements for ethical approval have
been a force for good, and have directed the attention of research workers to issues which are genuinely important and
which should be intrinsic to the intellectual milieu of medical
investigation.

The bioethical movement is different. While the ethical movement has been largely concerned with normative ethics, the
bioethical movement is at least partly concerned with meta-
ethical views. Normative ethicists helped the medical profession
to develop what amounts to a code of behaviour, a list of com-
mandments or maxims which can be applied equally to policy
decisions and to individual events. The bioethical dimension is
more abstract. It deals with the ontology, epistemology and
logical status of people's views on death and dying, their concepts of illness and suffering, the ownership of bodies before and
after death, the meaning and value of autonomy and quality of
life and many other fundamental issues and attitudes which
should determine the way medicine should be practised in a
pluralist society which insists that respect for personal autonomy is a defining attribute. ('Ontology' is the branch of metaphysics concerned with the nature of existence.)

The first problem for bioethicists is the nature of society. The
second lies in the nature of ethical debate. Pluralism and respect
for autonomy are two of the pillars of Western society. Bioethicists can only work by consensus, and consensus can only be
reached by compromise. The formulation of the Oregon scheme
— in which the state legislature held public meetings around the
state to develop a consensus about levels of basic medical care —
has shown that a measure of consensus can be reached in a
moderate sized society,[3,4] but consensus is not unanimity, and
discussions involving many people are bound to produce a dis-
affected minority at best, or a divided community at worst. A
committee agreement on a pattern of ethical behaviour and a set

of guiding moral values does not automatically translate into a set of precepts that will appeal to all members of a profession.

Ethics and laws

Furthermore, as chapter 7 showed, ethical guidelines cannot be enforced. Modern Western societies lack a secular moral authority with enough force to ensure the observation of its moral rules.[5] Learned colleges may rescind diplomas, medical boards may deregister and hospital authorities may withdraw privileges for serious breaches of ethical codes, but these are legal or quasi-legal sanctions which remove the issue from the purely moral domain. Ethics deals with conceptions of good and the fulfilment of voluntary obligations by autonomous individuals. Once there is a legal reason to follow a certain line of behaviour, the compulsion is quite different. What may have begun as a moral precept has become a law, and the relationship of individuals to the law is different from their relationship to their own conscience.

There is another important point. The intrusion of the law may involve another ethical dimension. Kantians, as discussed in chapter 7, presuppose that people acting according to the dictates of their own consciences should be acting according to Kant's famous categorical imperative.[6] Those who act from fear that the law may catch them, act according to a hypothetical imperative. They may also face another ethical dilemma on a different level if they believe strongly that an action contrary to law may be an action providing the best outcome. Doctors who establish a deep rapport with dying patients may agree completely when the patients urge the shortening of their life to end suffering and indignity, yet fear to act because they fear the legal consequences. Thus, the law removes the act from the purely moral universe, but creates another dimension of ethical problems. A further law that might deal with the new ethical problem presumably creates yet another level of ethical difficulty, and the process leads to an infinite regress. The law, therefore, probably cannot solve the unresolved issues that emerge from ethical debate, and the necessity to insist on the central importance of ethics in the definition and behaviour of professionalism remains paramount.

There is a further ontological point of importance. A particular practice in any medical institution may proceed for years without criticism or thought, posing no ethical problem. One day, however, someone may note weaknesses in the practice and register their concern. From the moment concern is expressed an ethical problem exists, and it continues to exist until the issue is resolved. There are probably countless ethical issues not yet identified in every medical institution. When an ethical concern is registered an ethical issue comes into being, and to satisfy the ethical imperative of the bioethics committee demands that the ethical issues be examined promptly, and that advice and ethical judgment be elaborated and promulgated to all concerned. Since these are moral issues, all those involved in the issue concerned need to know what is at stake so that they can formulate their own views in an autonomous fashion and determine their own stance and relationship to the matters under discussion. The previous *status quo* cannot continue, because attitudes and concerns have surfaced which must inevitably define new liberties, new constraints, new relationships with the law and new relationships between responsible staff. This doctrine of promulgation seems fundamental to the functioning of a bioethics committee.

Matters of principle

A hypothetical example may help. A cardiac unit at a major teaching hospital conducts sophisticated investigations for cardiac arrhythmias. It has achieved a world-wide reputation for its work, and its caseload is heavy. Its members have developed the practice of using heavy sedation to minimise the discomfort of the unpleasant manipulations that are routinely used. Patients are essentially unconscious during the whole procedure, but there is no anaesthetist available to monitor patients during the period of heavy sedation. The estimated mortality of the heavy sedation technique is 1 in 750. The cumulative mortality among the patients being studied increases with the time between first identification and the time of the study, and will reach 5% by three months. Five studies are carried out each week in four sessions, and there is a three week wait on average for each patient. The three week wait is associated with a risk of death of 1 in 375.

The director of anaesthetics at the hospital is told what is happening in the cardiac department, and notifies the head of the cardiac unit and the general superintendent that he cannot condone such heavy sedation without anaesthetic monitoring. He is, however, only able to provide anaesthetic monitoring for two of the four sessions each week because his budget has been cut, and he cannot recruit more anaesthetists. The director of cardiology points out that halving the number of sessions will double the waiting time and double the mortality on the waiting list to about 1 in 180. The director of anaesthetics insists that he cannot ethically allow the present practice to continue, and that it is within the power of the director of cardiology to reduce still further the very small risk of death from the sedation technique. The director of cardiology insists that she cannot ethically reduce the number of sessions since the heavy sedation technique has a low mortality, significantly lower than the mortality associated with doubling the waiting times for the studies. The general superintendent writes to the presidents of the respective learned colleges. Both presidents respond by saying that they cannot condone heavy sedation without anaesthetic supervision.

The situation is now thoroughly unsatisfactory. The director of cardiology points to the department's new ethical dilemma. Cardiac lists will be curtailed, and waiting times will soon double.

She insists that, on ethical grounds, she cannot accept the responsibility for the inevitable increase in mortality, and threatens to explain to patients that the general superintendent has introduced cutbacks which reduce the availability of medical care. The director of anaesthetics remains firm. On ethical grounds, he cannot condone anything short of the best practice. The learned colleges express their total commitment to the maintenance of standards. The general superintendent faces the dilemma of choice between the deontologically 'correct' decision to insist on optimum practice in an ideal world, and the utilitarianist 'correct' decision to maximise benefit to the community of patients with serious arrhythmias. Part of the problem resides in the conflicting moral bases of the various protagonists.

How might a bioethics committee approach this problem? Without making the decision analysis data specific, the general principles underlying the disagreement are these. A particular practice which is less than optimal allows a highly valued and effective service to reach the maximum number of people. The suboptimal practice is associated with a small risk of death, a risk which is smaller than that caused by the natural history of the untreated medical problem. Optimising the faulty practice will reduce the availability of the good service and will lead to a significant increase in suffering and death. The bioethics committee might start by considering the ethical issues in a formal manner.

What might the balance of good be under the doctrine of beneficence and non-maleficence? A utilitarian or consequentialist will say that the balance of risks clearly favours the *status quo*. Reducing the number of diagnostic sessions by 50% will significantly reduce the potential good. It would be better, in that view, to accept that in the real world of financial and personnel shortages there has to be a balance of risks, and that this balance cannot be reduced to something vanishingly small. A deontologist will tend to disagree. There are higher moral values than these. For a learned profession to survive, let alone thrive, it

113

must adopt absolute standards and adhere to them. How else can trust persist between patients and doctors?

Examination of the issue under the doctrine of autonomy is illuminating. The autonomy of the cardiologists has been challenged by the intervention of autonomous others and by the corporate morality of professional bodies. Obviously, professional autonomy must be limited in order to maintain standards and prevent corrupt and dangerous practice. No one, however, has considered anyone else's autonomy so far. The issue can be presented to patients and their families, perhaps in the reasonably comprehensible form of a decision tree. It is certainly reasonable to ask patients to help, and to declare their attitudes to risk. The choice is clear: the small risk of a sedation-related death or the larger risk of waiting longer so that anaesthetic supervision will be available. The nursing and technical staff are as autonomous as the doctors and patients, and they too should have a say about their relationships to the moral issues. Their misgivings about being involved in the *status quo* or its proposed alternative need to be examined and respected.

What of the principle of justice? If the waiting lists increase in length, a new pressure will arise. Those who can pay will urge a transfer to a private system, in which anaesthetists are likely to be available. This rich–poor division may not be just in the deontological sense, but to the utilitarian there is less of a problem. After all, those who can afford private care are better off than they were, and those who must remain within the public system are no worse off, and may actually benefit because the wealthy are dealt with elsewhere and the waiting list within the public system is shortened. Deontologists may see this issue quite differently.

The stances taken by the various parties in this example depend largely on the fourth fundamental of ethical practice — that of professional competence, and the ideal of best possible practice. The anaesthetists respect the cardiologists as cardiologists, as professional ethics prescribes, but cannot condone their activities as anaesthetists. The learned colleges in turn perceive their responsibility to protect the paradigms of good practice as a deontological categorical imperative. Their reputations depend on the clarity of their views and on their adherence to an ideal. Once confronted by such an issue, they are bound to respond by expressing that ideal as the only principle that they can endorse. The cardiologists, on the other hand, can point to the very low mortality achieved in practice, and to their skills in cardiovascular resuscitation based on a profound everyday knowledge of cardiac and vascular functioning in health and disease. Their competence is based on experience and demonstrated by the statistics of their practice. They adopt a utilitarian approach.

Argument from different premises

The difficulty has been created by the differences in moral theory unconsciously adopted by the various protagonists. Ethical teaching in most medical curricula is relatively superficial, and seldom equips medical graduates to understand the gravity of the issues that constantly arise in medical practice. In medicine, those who argue about issues like the one in the example adopt the deontological or utilitarian stance as it suits them (and sometimes shift ground during the discussion as it suits them), without recognising that the conflict that follows is unresolvable unless there is a philosophically messy but very practical compromise.

Philosophers and doctors alike recognise that it is sometimes easier to argue a strong (or extreme) case than it is to defend a weak one. Medical people tend to adopt a strongly deontological or a strongly utilitarian view in their ethical disputes, but the same people may move between the two extremes when defending the same position. In the example, the apparently utilitarian cardiologists may insist that saving human life and improving its qualities are ethical matters that must transcend all others. In making this claim, they would be recognising that deontological

115

views exist, and must be respected. Indeed, all utilitarian thinking has to have a deontological base, since it begins with the agreement that qualities such as human happiness and welfare are paramount. Similarly, deontologists have to consider the consequences of their actions, and decide whether their rules should apply in this particular case. As Rawls[7] said: 'All ethical doctrines worth our attention take consequences into account in judging rightness.' In medical ethics, regardless of the moral theory, each decision must have a teleological component — what is best for the patient, what is best for society and whether patient autonomy can be conserved or restored.

By this stage it should be clear that the bioethics committee may have provided some interesting insight into the nature of the problem and the intractable disagreements between the various parties, but there is no advice that might lead to a resolution. Medicine is wholly practical, and practitioners, when faced with a dilemma, seek a resolution which will enable action. Philosophers may sympathise with this requirement, but a bioethics committee faces a problem if it assumes or is required to adopt any legislative functions. It can only define the issues and advise an executive committee. Legislative decisions must be made by a different body. Once there is a legal or quasi-legal requirement to act in a particular way, the issue has been removed from the ethical domain, and a new potential ethical issue has been created as health professionals confront any potential conflict between their own ethical commitments and the new legal requirement. A hospital or health service investing in a bioethics advisory group must therefore define and limit its expectations for the scope of the committee's activities. It must expect a high level of scepticism from health professionals whose training emphasises the value of concrete decision-making, and whose expectations will include solutions to problems that inhibit practice and research. Therefore, although a bioethics committee can provide insight and advice, the legislative responsibility must remain with executive groups within the organisation.

The wide reflective equilibrium

It is clear that a bioethics committee cannot deliver consistent advice unless the conflict between deontological and utilitarian views can be resolved. Committees consisting entirely of deontologists or utilitarians will not be acceptable in a pluralist society. In medical ethics, there must be a shift from strict adherence to one of the classical moral grounds to a position which allows advice that may guide action. Everyone holds moral values — some values more or less intuitively, others evolved out of experience, teaching or learning. Reasonable and socially integrated people can usually agree on the justice or rightness of some courses of action. With that background, medical ethicists have some hope of working within what Daniels[8] called a wide reflective equilibrium. This term refers to a coherent system of ethics which derives its force from accepting moral intuitions and judgments in relation to practical experience. It suggests that it must be possible to generate acceptable moral principles, which may have a utilitarian or deontological bias. It also holds that such a system must be sustained by background theories concerning humanity and society, such as the social contract theory of Rawls.[7] Daniels[8] wrote from the point of view of a deontologist, but the English utilitarian philosopher Hare has proposed a similar model.[9]

Although the wide reflective equilibrium may seem too indefinite and altogether too far removed from the practical decision-making of clinical medicine, it has advantages as the basis of an ethical system for medicine. This ideal has been very well expressed by Wulff, Andur Pedersen and Rosenberg[10] when they wrote:

All doctors who have seriously tried to analyse the ethical foundation of their decision will have to admit that it is often difficult to reconcile their intuitions with their various duties, eg. their duty to choose that decision which has the best consequences for the patient, the duty to respect the patient's autonomy, and, especially if they are working in a national health service with a fixed budget, the duty to ensure that everybody gets a fair deal . . . A system of medical ethics cannot be viewed in isolation, but must be harmonized with the general norms and values of that particular society. Doctors sometimes forget this and believe that international codes of ethics express ethical 'truths' which are internationally valid just like scientific truths . . . such codes are much too vague to offer guidance in clinical practice, or they reflect the moral beliefs in a particular cultural setting, usually Europe and North America . . . In spite of all these difficulties, we maintain that it is the ultimate goal of ethical studies to establish a wide reflective equilibrium, just as it is the ultimate goal of science to establish the full truth, but we must also admit that in both cases the goal is unattainable.

The equilibrium in practice

We now turn back to the problem with which this discussion began. Is it possible, from within the wide reflective equilibrium, to conceive an ethically acceptable advice that might produce a solution to the hypothetical example? Preserving the *status quo*, with cardiologists administering heavy sedation in the face of anaesthetic criticism and opposition, is not tenable. Once the issue has emerged as an issue with substance (in this case confirmed by the opinions of the learned colleges), the hospital administration can no longer condone its continuation. The legal and moral objections would be both serious and substantial. To conform to the requirements of the anaesthetists, reducing the number of studies but providing anaesthetic monitoring, will solve one moral (and potential legal) problem, but obviously creates another. More people will suffer for longer, and more will die. Furthermore, obedience to the deontological judgment of the anaesthetic group excludes the autonomous rights of a disadvantaged group of ill people to make their own choice, based on their own assessment of the balance of risk.

No solution can be found until all parties abandon strict deontological or strict utilitarian grounds for their arguments, and adopt the wider view. There is a problem: it has been defined, enunciated and registered as a problem. The purpose of medicine is the preservation or restoration of well-being. How can this purpose be preserved in the dispute? The risk of the heavy sedation technique is small. The dispute has arisen because of a matter of principle, not because of a series of documented disasters. Now that the dispute is notified, the legal implications have changed. A disaster occurring after definition of the problem could be said in court to have occurred because the hospital administration was negligent in not intervening, and because the cardiologists were callously indifferent to individual safety. Neither of these accusations would be 'true', because they would impute motives that were not present.

If all parties can agree that patient welfare is paramount, that professional competence is a central issue, that patient autonomy must be respected and that the ethical intuitions and beliefs of the concerned health professionals deserve respect, then a solution must be available. The anaesthetists could, for example, offer to arrange a short course on heavy sedation and the necessary monitoring for medical and nursing staff, and arrange an accreditation system which would register their satisfaction with the knowledge and skills of those involved. The cardiologists could examine their data to determine markers that may define a particularly high-risk group, and schedule studies for those patients at times when anaesthetic monitoring was available. This kind of compromise may solve the logistic problems and go some way to resolving the ethical dilemma, which is totally bound to the practical issue of providing service. But there are further responsibilities, which follow the identification of the problem.

The promulgation of information and the explanation of the moral and practical issues are fundamental to the process of applied ethics. Informed consent is accepted as a necessity in the doctor–patient transaction. It is just as important to the activities of all health professionals faced with a decision which may have quasi-legal force, but which began as an ethical issue. The final decision — made by an executive committee, not the bioethical group — may still clash with individual moral intuitions and beliefs, and the autonomy of the health professionals then becomes a matter of major ethical importance.

It is self-evident that ethical argument cannot lead to a single truth. At best, it can illuminate. At its worst, it can confuse matters and paralyse action. At the same time, its importance cannot really be denied. Although logical positivists and emotivists have decried ethical thinking and ethical argument, morals and ethics provide the sole insight into Socrates' question: 'How should a man live?' As Williams[11] wrote: 'It is not a trivial question, Socrates said: what we are talking about is how one should live. Or so Plato reports him . . . Plato thought that philosophy could answer the question. Like Socrates, he hoped that one could direct one's life, if necessary redirect it, through an understanding that was distinctively philosophical — that is to say, general and abstract, rationally reflective, and concerned with what can be known through different types of inquiry.' Inquiry in medicine, as we have seen, usually produces probabilities rather than certainties. Uncertainty adds to the difficulties of ethical thinking, as it does to the processes of communication between doctors and patients. Thus, the issue of informed consent will be discussed next, as that is the point where issues of ethics and communication most obviously meet.

NOTES

1. World Medical Association Declaration of Helsinki, reproduced in Campbell A, Gillett G, Jones G. Practical medical ethics. Auckland: Oxford University Press, 1992:162–6.
2. Campbell A, Gillett G, Jones G. Practical medical ethics. Auckland: Oxford University Press, 1992:82.
3. Liu JT-Y. Oregon con: Oregon's experiment: just another Medicaid cutback. American College of Surgeons Bulletin 1993; 78–3:8–14.
4. Thorne JI. Oregon pro: as the nation waits, Oregon moves forward. American College of Surgeons Bulletin 1993; 78–3: 8–14.

5. Engelhardt HT Jr. National health care policy: the moral issues. American College of Surgeons Bulletin 1993; 78-4:10-14.
6. Kant I. Fundamental principles of the metaphysics of ethics, 10th edn, Abbott TK, trans. London: Longmans, Green & Co, 1940.
7. Rawls J. A theory of justice. Oxford: Oxford University Press, 1972.
8. Daniels N. Reflective equilibrium and Archimedean points. Canadian Journal of Philosophy 1980; 10:83-103.
9. Hare RM. Moral thinking. Its levels, method and point. Oxford: Clarendon Press, 1984.
10. Wulff HR, Pedersen SA, Rosenberg R. Philosophy of medicine — an introduction, 2nd edn. Oxford: Blackwell Scientific Publications, 1990:172-202.
11. Williams B. Ethics and the limits of philosophy. London: Fontana/Collins, 1985.

9

Autonomy, Logic, Hermeneutics and Informed Consent

Many bioethicists regard respect for autonomy as a central principle in determining how doctors should act both in medical practice and in clinical research. Informed consent is regarded as perhaps the most important concept flowing from the primacy of the doctrine of autonomy.[1-3] Although most would agree that the concept is important, understanding of it is imperfect, and there are many and conflicting views of its nature and its procedures. These uncertainties exist mainly because of a confusion between the institutional or legal concept (which requires certain procedures to be observed as evidence that informed consent has been given by patients), and the ethical concept of informed consent as an autonomous authorisation to proceed with treatment or to enter a clinical trial. Indeed, Katz[3] holds that courts and medical institutions have allowed informed consent to fail as a doctrine, because legal consent may leave the real requirements for autonomous authorisation unsatisfied. Others have recommended abandoning the term 'informed consent', using 'informed choice' or 'informed request' instead to emphasise the active role of the patient.[4] Nevertheless, the term persists, both in ethical and legal discussions. The ethical principles underlying informed consent apply to both human research and clinical intervention. At the simplest level (a general practitioner

122

consultation for renewal of a prescription or a straightforward examination for life assurance), authorisation is implied by the consultative process, which allows physical examination without specific consent. There is similar agreement that there is no need to lose time in seeking specific authorisation when a young, seriously ill patient presents to a hospital unconscious after an accident. The theory and practice of informed consent are at their most challenging when a major intervention with uncertain consequences is proposed for a life-threatening illness suffered by a competent patient. Most of what is said in this discussion concerns these more complex and demanding clinical situations, in which formal informed consent must be sought before treatment begins.

Fundamentals of informed consent

Beauchamp and Childress offered a clear analysis of contemporary attitudes to informed consent.[1] In brief, they listed five elements:
1. competence of the patient to understand the issues and to give consent;
2. disclosure of the relevant issues by the doctor;
3. an understanding of the issues by the patient;
4. a voluntary choice by the patient;
5. an autonomous authorisation by the patient for the treatment to be administered or for the terms of the clinical trial to be observed.

Beauchamp and Childress stressed that competence is indispensable to fully informed consent. It has been defined in terms of the subject's 'ability to perform a task',[5] a definition which immediately introduces problems of relative competence and differing standards of competence. It is also argued that different levels of competence are required for decisions involving greater or less complexity.[6] Beauchamp and Childress[1] suggested that a ranking of incompetencies might be possible

using the following scale, with 1 as the most profound incompetence and 7 the least serious:
1. inability to express preference or choice;
2. inability to understand one's situation;
3. inability to understand disclosed information;
4. inability to give a reason;
5. inability to give a rational reason, though having some supporting reasons;
6. inability to give a risk–benefit related reason though able to give some supporting reasons;
7. inability to give a reasonable decision, judged by the 'reasonable person' standard.

Competence is clearly a difficult issue, particularly when age, mental disability, psychiatric illness and altered consciousness diminish or take away the ability to make an autonomous decision. Furthermore, clinical impressions about competence are unreliable, and a variety of structured tests may be needed to determine the level at which autonomous decisions can truly take place.[7,8]

Few people these days would argue with the need for doctors to disclose all the relevant facts about what they propose to do, whether in conventional treatment or as part of a clinical trial. The term 'relevant', however, is imprecise. Once again, there are standards of disclosure, but no agreement on the preferred standard.[1] The 'professional practice' standard is commonly used, both in ethical and legal discussion. The 'standard' here refers to the accepted practice of the medical profession at the time. The 'reasonable person' standard suggests that disclosure should be comprehensive enough to satisfy a reasonable person. These standards have been used for many years, but are being progressively replaced by the subjective standard, which posits that disclosure should be tailored as far as possible to the individual to whom the disclosure will be made. This is clearly a demanding standard to meet, since it could only be satisfied if doctors examine patients' biographies in more detail than may be possible in practice.

Unfortunately, there are practical difficulties because these standards are necessarily vague and undefined. While they may suggest guidelines for ethical action, the courts may not accept that actions fulfil the guidelines if a legal case hinges on an ethical matter, such as the adequacy of the disclosure within the process of informed consent. Studies of living donors who have given kidneys to relatives with kidney failure have suggested that full disclosure did not necessarily translate into full understanding.[9,10] Other studies have shown that full disclosure to cancer patients in structured interviews affected patient perceptions of the proposed treatment or trial.[11] Patients to whom full disclosure was made had a better understanding of treatment and its side-effects, but were less willing to be randomised in a study, and demonstrated significantly higher levels of anxiety.

Disclosure will only have meaning if it is understood by patients. Indeed, understanding can be seen as more important conceptually than detailed disclosure.[12] This view emphasises the potential division between understanding and explanation, a problem that occupies a major place in modern hermeneutic thinking.[13] It is also important to appreciate that patients who have given satisfactory informed consent commonly forget details, such as the name or the purpose of an operation, within a few months.[14] Ethically, this may not matter, but it may become a key issue for the legal system. These complexities emphasise the values of hermeneutics (understanding human communication) in the process of obtaining informed consent. Doctors and patients must both try to understand the impact of their different biographies and ideologies before true discourse can take place. In this context, Habermas's concepts of discourse ethics[15] (an ethical system which derives its force from discussion of ethical issues to a point of agreement among those with legitimate interest in a contentious issue, rather than from purely deontological or utilitarian principles) and of ideology critique[16] (a process of deliberate examination of the ideological commitments of the parties to a discourse, so that all sides can appreciate the values and the meaning of concepts that emerge during the discourse) seem useful in delineating the agenda for doctors and patients in reaching a proper informed consent.

Under the doctrine of autonomy, informed consent is faulty unless it is voluntarily given. There are three ways in which true voluntariness can be impaired: coercion, manipulation or persuasion.[1]

Coercion may take many forms, but all depend on clinicians enforcing their preference for treatment by threats which they can make because of their power of superior knowledge, and the relative weakness of ill patients. Clinicians who say that they will refuse to take further responsibility for treatment unless patients enter a particular clinical trial use coercion.

Persuasion is the process by which clinicians may change patients' minds by force of argument. If the argument is valid and the clinicians' attitude is governed by a genuine desire to benefit patients (the principle of beneficence), persuasion may be a legitimate part of the process of obtaining informed consent. If, for example, a surgeon persuades a 21-year-old with polyposis coli to have a colectomy because he knows that within a few years she will develop invasive adenocarcinoma of the colon, he is probably doing the patient a service, although she may have no symptoms at the time of the consultation.

Manipulation is neither rational persuasion nor coercion, and perhaps most frequently involves the selective presentation of data. A surgeon who has a new method of treating liver metastases may say that this new treatment is very promising, and that 32% of patients are responding favourably to it in the short term. She may manipulate the patient into entering a trial by withholding the information that there are other methods of palliative treatment with known long-term results and that the new treatment involves considerable discomfort and restriction of activity by comparison with the established methods.

The final step in the process of informed consent comes when patients agree to authorise clinicians to carry out the treatment, or consent to enter a trial. It has been shown that patient attitudes to authorisation can be influenced by the way information is presented during the act of disclosure in a clinical setting,[17] just as information alters perceptions of the consequences of entering a clinical trial.[11] After a structured interview, patients are less likely to sign a consent form, but are more likely to join doctors in the decision-making process. Katz[12] said that informed consent is indeed best conceptualised in this way, as a transaction of mutual decision-making by patients and doctors.

Ethics, law and informed consent

The confusion commonly encountered in medical ethics between legal and moral requirements is probably worst in this area of informed consent. A sharp distinction needs to be drawn between the ethical content of informed consent (which is concerned with the good that it brings) and the institutional form (which is concerned with its legal implications), but the distinction is commonly ignored.[1,18] The confusion that follows unsettles both doctors and patients. The confusion inevitably arises when people try to argue from radically different premises: from the position of a deontological universal categorical imperative ('informed consent is a good in itself') on the one hand and from a utilitarian relative (legal) imperative ('I may be sued if I don't get you to sign this paper') on the other. The moral bases for these are different, and the legal imperative raises a whole set of ethical problems by diverting attention from the essentially moral dimension of the process of seeking informed consent. More specifically, the adversarial model followed in countries with law derived from the British system exaggerates the separation of legal from moral issues, pushing the informed consent issue further into the institutional arena. The need to act defensively in the matter of informed consent can readily override any spontaneous or learned sensitivity to the vulnerability of sick people and their need to understand their illness and the potential for healing.

The extent of this problem has been emphasised by an analysis of medico-legal cases. Hawkins and Paterson examined the issues underlying a series of legal actions against doctors and health facilities.[19] They documented a failure of communication — amounting to a failure of informed consent — in 27% of the cases. They advised readers to seek ways to improve their methods of seeking informed consent, but saw the main issue as medico-legal, to be approached by improving consent forms. It seems unlikely that scrupulous attention to the legalities will satisfy patients who seem to want more sympathetic discourse and a recognition that the real point of informed consent is that it should recognise their individuality and autonomy.[20]

The prominence of the legal element in the issue of informed consent reflects in some part the medical devotion to the biopositivist model. Positivism concludes that there is no point in dealing with anything that is not self-evidently true, or that cannot be examined objectively by empirical methods. The precept that 'It is morally good that patients should make autonomous decisions to authorise medical treatment' has less empirical content than one that says 'A doctor who fails to obtain written consent to treatment is likely with probability p to be sued if something goes wrong.' People who have been educated to sustain the biopositivist model will certainly feel that the second statement has more meaning than the first. It is unlikely, however, that the positivist approach will resolve the unsettled issues that interfere with the doctor–patient relationship. Resolution, if it comes, will follow the use of the biohumane model instead of the biopositivist, because only by working within the real function of the principle of autonomy and its derivative principle of informed consent can the very real concerns of patients be allayed. As we shall see, neither logic nor the law provide satisfactory alternatives to the process of discourse.

It is important to stress the destructive influence of the division within medicine between the reductionist conception that illness is best understood by tracking disease to increasingly fundamental levels of the organ, the cell and the gene, and the holistic conception that what makes humanity unique is something more than the sum of the fundamental parts. If doctors did not have an elevated view of humanity as being human, there would be no edifice erected for the maintenance or restoration of health, autonomy and quality of life. If all that mattered really was the health of the liver, there would be no priority attached to healing the human liver, rather than that of a dog or cat, when it was sick. Hepatologists happily use the rat liver as a 'model', but justify their existence and the existence of their research programs by stressing the potential for finding ways to ensure the function of humans as holistic structures, with apparently unique cognitive and moral dimensions. Informed consent should emerge naturally from this implicit belief in the unique status of humanity and the unique place of medicine in the welfare of individuals and populations. Constructive thought about informed consent is not possible outside this conception. If the law has to be involved (and I am sure that it must), no one should consider that the solutions to the important ethical problems will be found in legislation. We will examine the problems with applying logic shortly.

Particular problems of the controlled trial

Obtaining informed voluntary authorisation for treatment for medical disability is hard enough even when there is only one preferred treatment. Obtaining consent that is truly 'informed' for a controlled trial is even more difficult. Levine[21] pointed out that an honest hypothesis demands that treatments A and B do not allow a scientifically valid reason for predicting that one treatment is better than the other. Moreover, there can be no therapy C known to be better than A or B, unless there is good reason to reject C or patients voluntarily refuse C. Thus, it would be quite unethical to compare blood-letting (A) with leeching (B) in the treatment of pneumonia, even though they were once recognised treatments, because doctors know that penicillin (C) is almost always effective. The restriction imposed by strict experimental protocols may deprive patients of the 'good of personal care'. The negotiation may also steer patients away from palliative care, which might have been chosen if a trial was not in progress. Freireich[22] used the notion of sick clinicians to question the morality of the controlled trial. Sick clinicians, in Freireich's experience, do not seek out the best controlled trial, but the best clinician for their personal care.

Cultural differences

To compound these difficulties, we must recognise that Anglo-American values are not the only ones that need to be considered. There is evidence of a profound relativism in the ethical literature. In France, for example, Bernard enunciated the view that knowledge expansion is so important in medical science that it should precede respect for individuals and their liberty.[23] In Japan, Hoshino stressed that patients' rights to refuse information must be respected — in Hoshino's (translated) words, we must allow anyone to place a 'veto on their own rights'.[24]

These differences are also important within pluralistic and multicultural societies. People of different religious beliefs, cultural backgrounds and values mingle in large cities in many parts of the world. This very major problem for medical understanding is not within the scope of this book: it would take an entire book to examine the subject in depth.

Critique of the concept of autonomy

The case has been made that autonomy is impaired to some degree by every illness.[25] There may, therefore, be reasons to seek other justifications for seeking informed consent than a simple appeal to full autonomy. Wear[26] felt that current bio-ethical scholarship and pedagogy have too little correlation with the realities and variables of clinical medicine. Any worthwhile use of the concept of autonomy must be linked to clinical factors and will need to be heavily modified if it is to achieve practical force. Since all sick people have experienced some loss of autonomy, the medical task is to restore as much autonomy as possible.[25] Unsought paternalism that reduces autonomy still further is, in this perspective, the greatest wrong that doctors can impose. There are thus very fundamental reasons for confirming that all medical decisions need to be made with the patients' concurrence or implied concurrence, and should aim to improve or conserve the presenting level of autonomy. Observing even this simple principle is more difficult than it sounds, particularly when serious and life-threatening illness has to be discussed. The anxieties and deep wishes of patients may make understanding the medical disclosure almost impossible. Further, the patients may have worst fears about an outcome — death under anaesthesia, blindness, a colostomy, a diagnosis of cancer — which depend on the (often secret) biography of them and their family, and which may not be discussed because the issues are neither mentioned nor suspected. A short formal analysis reveals how precarious the basis of informed consent may be.

The logic of informed consent

In this short and formal analysis, x is the individual patient with diagnosis F, X is the class of all patients with diagnosis F, and G is the (single) desired outcome of treatment P appropriate for diagnosis F which will follow with probability p.

When x approaches her doctor with a problem, x wants her particular symptoms and signs diagnosed. When the diagnosis F is confirmed, x expects P as the 'best' treatment, and expects a desirable outcome G (preservation of life, enhanced quality of life, restoration of autonomy) because she believes that the science of medicine has produced treatment P to achieve outcome G in the whole class of patients X with diagnosis F. This belief is rooted in the patient's understanding of medicine as a 'scientific' discipline with access to the same kind of determinism as astronomy or physics. Since patient x belongs to the class of patients X, she expects the anticipated good result G rather than the alternative unsatisfactory outcome $\sim G$.

For the doctor, however, the ground rules are quite different. Certainly, x belongs to the class X, but the results of treatment P can only be predicted from inductive inference based on empirical observation. The desired outcome G is not deterministic, but stochastic (probabilistic), and there is no way for the doctor to be absolutely sure that the agreed 'best' treatment P will produce outcome G in this particular patient. All that the doctor can do is to quote objective probabilities modified by his own subjective probabilities which express to some extent the dynamics of his belief systems, and leave the patient with a final uncertainty about the outcome of treatment.

This very simple analysis of a complex matter shows that the end-point of the consultation may be profoundly unsatisfactory for both parties. The patient's notion that all patients with diagnosis F should do well with treatment P is probably based on a folk appreciation of medicine as a science, and of science as dealing in determinism. Views of this kind have been often promulgated by the lay press and television, which do much to shape folk images of science and medicine. Even though the doctor may also feel that medicine is a science, he cannot command the determinism that would satisfy the patient. In the end, both doctor and patient arrive back at the point which motivated the original consultation: a patient who does not know whether she personally (as a unique individual) will be 'cured' or not. Understandably, it also often leaves the patient asking why there is no precision when there is so much science. Whatever way we choose to examine this process, it is clear that genuinely informed consent must be rare in a situation of any complexity because the requirements of the patient may not be satisfied by the ultimate uncertainty of the doctor's knowledge.

The problem therefore cannot be solved by logic, nor by legislation which defines burdens of responsibility for individual doctors and medical institutions. If there is any resolution, it is likely to come from a hermeneutic approach, from finding a way to communicate the realities of treatment outcomes and the potential risks of any treatment — that is, by transferring it from the institutional domain back to the ethical domain of good communication where it properly belongs. But how do doctors communicate to patients the consequences of a decision to choose one treatment in preference to another, when there are probable or possible benefits to be balanced against probable or possible risks?

We will use the example of a patient with a serious illness which unmistakably threatens to end the patient's life within the next two years. A solitary metastasis has been detected in the left liver six months after the patient has undergone right hemi-colectomy for carcinoma of the colon. The diagnosis has been proven, and doctor and patient are at the stage of discussing options for treatment. We will simplify the discussion by assuming that the doctor's previous experience convinces her that surgical removal of an apparently solitary metastasis is the 'best' treatment that can be offered, because 27% of patients treated in this way survive more than two years and other methods of treatment do not influence life span, although they may improve the quality of residual life. Surviving beyond two years is the outcome that the patient desires. The doctor needs to obtain informed consent to either surgical removal or 'other methods of treatment'. This example has been greatly simplified for this analysis: commonly, a number of other options would be discussed. The complexity of obtaining informed consent increases rapidly as the number of choices increases. It is necessary to examine in hermeneutic terms what it is the patient needs to hear, and what the doctor is entitled to say while adhering to a notion of 'warranted assertibility' within a coherent structure of medical knowledge.[27]

In explaining with the purpose of creating understanding, we can extend Peirce's concept of community[28] into a thought experiment by invoking the model of two rooms each with a community of 100 people suffering from solitary liver metastases at time 0. The rooms are revisited two years from now. If all of those in room 1 had 'other treatment' ($\sim P$), we might find one or two people alive. In room 2, whose occupants underwent treatment by liver resection (P), we would find 27 still alive, even allowing for the dangers of treatment by liver resection. This is easier to visualise than the standard gamble,[29] easier to adapt to clinical reality than the marble drawing models, and it is easy enough to extend these community models to explain the risks of death-from-treatment and morbidity-from-treatment.

Some alternative doctrines

Fully informed consent is probably never attainable, since people have by definition lost some measure of autonomy and generally cannot be informed of the immense complexities of the biological processes involved, many of which remain unknown to doctors. In most instances, patients cannot have a realistic appreciation of something never experienced before. Pain is terrible at the time, but cannot really be remembered once it is over. Someone facing painful surgery can be warned about the pain, but cannot appreciate the experience before it happens. There are no words that will evoke physical pain, so a consent to a painful procedure is a consent to suffer whatever it is that constitutes severe pain. Professor George Wilson of Edinburgh wrote to James Young Simpson, the man who introduced chloroform for anaesthesia, about the experience of undergoing a Syme's amputation of one foot by Syme himself: 'Suffering so great as I underwent cannot be expressed in words, and thus fortunately cannot be recalled . . . I still recall with unwelcome vividness the spreading out of the instruments: the twisting of the tourniquet: the first incision: the fingering of the sawed bones: the sponge pressed on the flap: the tying of the blood vessels: the stitching of the skin: and the bloody dismembered limb lying on the floor.'[30] The idea of the agony is disturbing enough, but the pain remains beyond communication. It is quite common for patients to say how completely unprepared they were for the severity of the pain of an illness or operation. Similarly, the disability caused by the loss of a leg can be explained, but not understood until actually experienced. The same observations apply to the effects of long-term use of β-blockers, with the physical fatigue and leg-tiredness that reduce the quality of life and autonomy of action. Since these physical experiences cannot regularly be communicated in words, even by skilled communicators, the consent can only be partly informed. Since it is not logically possible to satisfy a patient with a fatal disease who is looking for a cure, it would be wise for clinicians to suggest some modifications to the precepts that guide the debate about informed consent.

1. *Informed advice to the level of individual competence.* There is both legal and moral force to this doctrine. The difficulty lies in knowing someone else's level of competence. The practical solution lies in holding as much discourse as doctor and patient require for the doctor (as discloser) to judge the appropriate level of disclosure. The onus must be on the doctor to make this judgment. Medical education needs to emphasise this responsibility and teach some of the appropriate skills.

2. *Advice to the point of individual satisfaction.* This doctrine has legal and moral components, but in this instance the responsibility must lie with the patient to define the extent to which information is essential and appropriate. As Hoshino[24] insisted, there are times when patients do not want further information, and that judgment must remain with the patients themselves. The law cannot insist on full disclosure if it is expressly rejected.

3. *Specific discourse on worst fears.* This particular doctrine is of recent origin, and follows the Australian High Court ruling in the case of *Rogers v Whittaker*.[31] In that case, Whittaker sought treatment for an eye complaint which had rendered her blind in one eye. She had a morbid fear of losing the sight in the

remaining eye, and was reassured that there was practically
no chance of that event. The condition of sympathetic ophthalmitis in which damage to the unoperated eye occurs,
probably from auto-immunity, was considered by the eye
surgeon to be so remote as to need no particular discussion.
Sympathetic ophthalmitis did in fact occur, with resulting
blindness in the remaining eye. The appeal judges found that
Rogers was wrong in not offering an extended discussion of
the patient's 'worst fear'. They overturned a long-standing
ruling that medical practice should be governed by the standards of reasonable practitioners at the time of the event,
holding instead that the courts should decide what was
reasonable. While their ruling relied on purely legal arguments, the doctrine clearly has moral as well as legal content.

4. *Bilateral responsibility*. It seems clear that the doctor must accept responsibility firstly for knowing what ought to be
disclosed, and secondly for assessing the competence of the
patient to understand that disclosure. It must also be accepted that the competent patient must accept responsibility
for defining the limits to the disclosure, and for agreeing to
limit the disclosure when he or she has reached a point of
satisfaction. This sharing of responsibility needs to become a
standard for the discourse which defines the ethical (rather
than legal) process of informed consent.

5. *Authorisation within accepted limits of autonomy*. Fully autonomous authorisation is probably unattainable from someone
who is ill. The illness limits autonomy in both obvious and
subtle ways. The process of consultation itself declares the
patient's desire to move from a position of impaired autonomy and diminished quality of life to a better state. This
petitionary state is inevitable. If it was not, there would be no
medical profession. This concept has both legal and moral
components.

6. *Proof of content*. The requirement that there be written evidence is a purely legal constraint. A signed consent form does
not guarantee a doctor or a hospital protection against legal

action, and it certainly does not ensure satisfaction for a patient. The signed form merely demonstrates that some process was followed to exchange information and answer questions. From a purely ethical view, the form does little to ensure the moral validity of the discourse which led to the signing of the form. Wrangling about the content of consent forms does not advance the debate on the ethical issues. In fact, by diverting attention from the fundamentally ethical content of the issue, it has probably done a great deal to inhibit profitable discourse.

There is a major need to refresh the debate about informed consent. The legal and institutional processes are unlikely to advance thinking, since they are concerned more with defence against legal actions, and diminish the real concern with patient benefit. Ethicists examining the problem cannot dissociate the argument from clinical realities, which involve stochastic causal mechanisms of great and unmeasured complexity. There can be no progress while the field is constrained by the strictures of adversarial law, which should not have a central role in the formulation of an ethic of communication. That ethic begins with the obligation of reasonable and skilled professionals to use their skills, including their communication skills, in the service of their patients. It may have been possible in earlier generations to practise paternalism and to defend it on the grounds of 'therapeutic privilege', but it is increasingly difficult to sustain that argument in the face of the stated desires of medical consumer groups. Tedious though clinicians may find the process, joint decision by patient and doctor after appropriate discourse is desirable. It is doubtful that this conclusion can ever be enforced by law or statute. There is no secular moral authority to enforce the ideal,[32] and no ethical code of practice will solve all the problems of the doctor–patient relationship.

The communication skills of medical graduates must be fostered and expanded, or misunderstandings will occur however meticulous and honourable the conduct of individual doctors. The path to improvement lies in education of undergraduates chosen for entry to medical faculties as much for their humane qualities as for their scientific skills. In the meantime, the bio-ethical debate needs to distinguish the ethical from the legal issues, and must include clinicians who have experienced the realities of medical encounters, and have the wisdom to recognise the primacy of communication in medicine and the eminence required to exert leadership without power. Above all, the debate requires faculties and learned colleges to commit themselves sincerely to recognising and promoting the validity of the biohumane model of medicine in research and practice. We will examine some of the implications of such a commitment in the next two chapters.

NOTES

1. Beauchamp TL, Childress JF. The principle of respect for autonomy. In: Principles of biomedical ethics. Oxford: Oxford University Press, 1989:67–119.
2. Meisel A, Roth L. What we do and do not know about informed consent. Journal of the American Medical Association 1981: 246:2473–7.
3. Katz J. Disclosure and consent. In: Milunsky A, Annas G, eds. Genetics and the law. New York: Plenum Press, 1980:122–8.
4. Campbell A, Gillett G, Jones G. Practical medical ethics. Auckland: Oxford University Press, 1992:21–3.
5. Culver CM, Gert B. Philosophy in medicine. Oxford: Oxford University Press, 1982:ch 3.
6. Abernathy V. Compassion, control, and decisions about competency. American Journal of Psychiatry 1984; 141:53–8.
7. Fitten LJ, Waite MS. Impact of medical hospitalisation on treatment decision-making capacity in the elderly. Archives of Internal Medicine 1990; 150:1717–21.
8. Fitten LJ, Lusky R, Hamann C. Assessing treatment decision-making capacity in elderly nursing home residents. Journal of the American Geriatric Society 1990; 38:1097–104.
9. Fellner CH, Marshall JR. Twelve kidney donors. Journal of the American Medical Association 1968; 206:2703–7.
10. Fellner CH, Marshall JR. Kidney donors — the myth of informed consent. American Journal of Psychiatry 1970; 126:1245.

11. Simes RJ, Tattersall MH, Coates AS, Raghavan D, Solomon HJ, Smartt H. Randomised comparison of procedures for obtaining informed consent in clinical trials of treatment for cancer. British Medical Journal, Clinical Research Edition 1986; 293:1065–8.
12. Katz J. The silent world of doctor and patient. New York: Free Press, 1984:86–7.
13. Ricoeur P. From text to action: essays in hermeneutics II. Blamey K, Thompson JB, trans. Evanston, Illinois: Northwestern University Press, 1991.
14. Lavelle-Jones C, Byrne DJ, Rice P, Cuschieri A. Factors influencing quality of informed consent. British Medical Journal 1993; 306:885–90.
15. Habermas J. Moral consciousness and communicative action. Lenhardt C, Nicholsen SW, trans. Cambridge: Polity Press, 1992.
16. Brand A. The force of reason: an introduction to Habermas' theory of communicative action. Sydney: Allen & Unwin, 1990.
17. Dawes PJ, O'Keefe L, Adcock S. Informed consent: using a structured interview changes patients' attitudes toward informed consent. Journal of Laryngology and Otology 1993; 107:775–9.
18. Lantos J. Informed consent: the whole truth for patients? Cancer 1993;72 (suppl):2811–5.
19. Hawkins C, Paterson I. Medicolegal audit in the West Midlands region: analysis of 100 cases. British Medical Journal Clinical Research Edition 1987; 295:1533–6.
20. Toombs SK. The meaning of illness. A phenomenological account of the different perspectives of physician and patient. Dordrecht: Kluwer Academic Publishers, 1992.
21. Levine RJ. Ethics of clinical trials. Do they help the patient? Cancer 1993;72 (suppl):2805–10.
22. Freireich EJ. The randomized clinical trial as an obstacle to clinical research. In: Delaney JP, Varco RL, eds. Controversies in surgery II. Philadelphia: WB Saunders, 1983:5–12.
23. Bernard J. Bioethics and knowledge. Nouvelle Revue Française d'Hematologie 1990; 32:377–85.
24. Hoshino K. Bioethical issues and principles in cancer treatment. Gan To Kagaku Ryoho 1992; 19:281–5.
25. Little JM. The potential contribution of autonomy to a calculus of clinical benefit. Theoretical Surgery 1994; 8:221–6.
26. Wear S. The irreducibly clinical character of bioethics. Journal of Medical Philosophy 1991; 16:53–70.
27. Smart JJC. Explanation — opening address. In: Knowles D, ed. Explanation and its limits. Cambridge: Cambridge University Press, 1990:1–20.

28. The American pragmatist philosopher Charles Peirce recognised that probability and chance could not be related in a meaningful way to individual persons or events. He introduced his notion of community to explain why probability remains a useful concept, because it described the outcomes that would be observed over time in a large enough group of events or people subject to natural processes or to specific interventions. He pointed out that this type of truth helped the understanding of events within a community, although it provided no certainty for the individuals within it. See Peirce CS. Doctrine of chances. Writings 1878; 3:281–2. Reprinted in: Houser N, Kloesel C, eds. The essential Peirce: selected philosophical writings, vol 1 (1867–1893). Bloomington and Indianapolis: Indiana University Press, 1992:142–54.

29. Clarke JR. A scientific approach to surgical reasoning. V. Patients' attitudes. Theoretical Surgery 1991; 6:166–76.

30. Quoted in Little JM. Amputation of the leg: a dull topic revisited. Medical Journal of Australia 1973; 2:442–5.

31. Rogers v Whittaker. High Court of Australia, 1992 67; 47–55.

32. Engelhardt HT Jr. National health care policy: the moral issues. American College of Surgeons Bulletin 1993; 78–4:10–14.

10

Text, Context and the Medical History

The communication involved in taking a patient's medical history is complex and frequently unsatisfactory, as chapter 9 showed. The process is taught at some length during medical courses, but it is the catechetical detail — the 'correct' questions and the acceptable answers — that preoccupies medical teachers, and the hermeneutic aspects are more or less ignored. This is unfortunate, because the unspoken and intersubjective part of medical histories is just as important as the formal questions and answers that are usually believed to comprise the essence of the exchange. Downie and Charlton[1] examined the value of education in the humanities as a way of increasing medical understanding of the patients' experience. Popper's concepts[2] were used to examine the general clinical process in some detail in chapter 2, and Toombs examined it from a phenomenological viewpoint.[3] Phenomenology requires us to divest the subject under investigation of its accepted meanings and values — to 'bracket' them — and to examine the pure phenomena that remain. Toombs did this by removing the medical values and meanings demanded by the biopositivist concept of health and disease, and examining the phenomena that remain for the patient experiencing the disturbances of illness. Concepts taken from linguistics (the scientific study of

141

language), semiology (the science which deals with communication by signs), discourse ethics (the philosophy of communitarian value setting) and modern hermeneutic philosophy (the philosophy of interpretation) can all help clinicians to understand the intricate dynamics of verbal communication within the clinical encounter.[4-6] First, we must look at some of the linguistic barriers to communication between doctors and patients.

The linguistics of medicine

Porter,[7] in a survey of the language of quacks,[8] wrote 'It is no accident that Apollo is god of both poetry and medicine, for the captivating power of song to move and soothe has always been seen to resemble the healing power of the word in sickness. From Greek 'incubation' therapy (in which the god spoke to the sick in dreams) through the bedside manner of the traditional clinician right up to Freud's psychoanalytical 'talking cure', language has ever been crucial to the profession and practice of medicine.'

There are four basic principles of sociolinguistics:[9]
1. different social groups use different varieties of language;
2. the same people use different varieties of language in different situations;
3. language reflects the society in which it is spoken;
4. language shapes the society in which it is spoken.

Burke[9] wrote 'The development of certain occupational languages . . . needs to be interpreted not only in a utilitarian way, as the creation of the technical terms for practical purposes, but also in a symbolic way, as the expression of a growing professional self-consciousness and of a growing distance from outsiders, such as the inhabitants of "Civvy Street".' Medicine has its own vocabulary of differentiation, focusing not on communicating with patients, but on communicating with fellow professionals.

A sociolinguistic examination of some key words is illuminating. 'Shock' and 'system' are two words in the linguistic space of attempted communication between patients and doctors. 'Shock' is a term commonly used by the general population. It may mean agitation at bad news, or distress at the experience of pain, among other things. It has bad connotations, but of a vague kind. This loosely descriptive but useful understanding of the word at the popular or 'folk' level contrasts sharply with the complex precision of its medical meaning. In medicine, 'shock' means a state of circulatory inadequacy with life-threatening implications. The medical usage is not 'more' nor 'less' correct than the non-medical meaning. The word did not begin as a medical term. Medicine took over a folk concept ('folk' means a word or concept that came from the common people, and has connotations of traditionalism, collective wisdom and sincerity).

The same applies to the word 'system' which, in lay terms, reflects a view of the holistic organisation of body function: 'she had such a shock that her system never recovered'. The medical profession's need for precision and its reductionist view, allow only the recognition of individual systems — the nervous system, the gastrointestinal system, the locomotor system and so on — each with its own special structure, functions and diseases. If doctors and patients are to understand one another, the potential incompatibility of the concepts underlying polysemes (words with multiple meanings) must be understood. This requires effort, tolerance and an awareness of the ways in which language works and linguistic worlds diverge.

Classification of disease

Direct communication is also impaired at times by the importance of the biomechanical model of disease. Medical education uses paradigmatic ('model') concepts of disease. It stresses typical cases, however rare these may be in practice. These paradigms are like Platonic forms, representing abstracts of 'perfect' disease.[10] Unfortunately, there is often a difference between the stylised disease and its manifestations in individuals. A person with 'atypical' abdominal pain may have gallstones, shown on an abdominal ultrasound. Removing the gall-bladder may not change the symptoms if they were actually due to irritable gut. Yet both doctor and patient feel that the existence of what is conceived to be pathological (structurally or functionally demonstrably abnormal) under the biomechanical model of disease must explain the pain, and that the pain will be cured by removing the gall-bladder.

This difference between the 'perfect' model, as it is taught, and the reality of a disease and its varying symptoms, lead to the concept of a 'good' history and a 'good' historian. A classical history and a clear demonstration of matching pathology, as we saw in chapter 2, are sufficiently rare for clinicians to use them as 'good' examples, fit for demonstrating to students. Such paradigm match is important, because it may reinforce an understanding of processes and mechanisms, but teachers need to stress that such a perfect match cannot and must not be expected in all cases with similar pathology.

Canguilhem examined the influence of ideologies on disease classification.[11,12] He made it clear that the medical reconstruction of the patients' narrative and its re-interpretation as medical history is also paradigmatic. Students of orthodox medicine are taught to take from the narrative those features that allow a logically coherent classification within the biomechanical model of illness. Students of other systems, such as homoeopathy or herbalism, learn to seek other information and to take different features from the patients' narrative. There have been attempts to compare homoeopathic and conventional treatments for the same illnesses, but the differences between the systems make it difficult for practitioners to agree on the nature of some of the diseases treated.[13] Beyond this clash of ideologies, there is a tension between 'scientific' knowledge (as conceived by orthodox practitioners) and other kinds of knowledge. The dominance of

British empiricism, with its pragmatic scepticism, at the expense of reflexive thought, intuition and the validity of personal experience, has benefited the science of medicine, but not its hermeneutics, a view eloquently elaborated by Cassell.[14] Whether doctors know it or not, there is always the possibility of confusion in consultations because of the linguistic habits of both doctors and patients, unintentionally used in the way they speak to each other. Each party attaches certain meanings to words and phrases and assumes that the meaning is understood by the other party — who may in fact hear the word or phrase and attach quite a different meaning to it. An example is the different meaning 'shock' holds for doctors and the general public.

Speech acts

Theories of speech acts have been elaborated by Austin[15] and Searle.[16] In analysing a speech act, people distinguish three levels at which the act may take place:

1. the level of the locutionary or propositional act (the act of saying);
2. the level of the illocutionary act (the force expressed in saying);
3. the level of the perlocutionary act (what we do by the fact that we speak).

If I say 'Bring me that book!', the locutionary act links you and a particular book together with an active verb (predicate). The illocutionary act is expressed by the fact that this is an order, not a statement, a wish or a promise. The perlocutionary act expresses the consequences of the speech act. My command may invoke a fear of disobeying, or anger at such an unreasonable demand. The perlocutionary act is largely confined to oral discourse, and this is relevant to speech acts in the medical history. Patients may strive to invoke pity in doctors, and doctors may want to make patients optimistic about the outcome of their illness. When the medical notes and the medical letter record this perlocutionary (emotional/unspoken) content, they do so by description and by interpretation which are distanced from the speech act and the subjective experience it came from.

This emphasises the relation of speaking to writing. Writing to some extent removes the text from the meaning of the author — in this case, from the meaning of the patient. In the medical context, doctors take the clinical narrative and create the text of the medical history in the form of medical notes and medical letters. The medical notes become the medical letter, and the reader — the referring doctor — puts the contents of the letter into their own context. Doctors may feel confident that their letters say exactly what they mean, and that they can have only one meaning. This is not true. Different educations, experiences and specialisations make the process of recontextualising more speculative and less uniform than we believe. It is notoriously difficult to reconstruct definitive and confident medical histories from historical narratives. We will probably never know the cause of Mozart's death, because the context of his illness was so drastically different from the context of illness as we understand it now, within our contemporary model of biopositivist explanation.[17]

We will return to this question of the alienating effect of text later in this chapter, but first we must take a semiological look at the basic signals that patients send during their individually unique consultations.

Why do people consult doctors?

People consult doctors because they perceive that there is something actually or potentially threatening the quality of their lives; because they fear that illness may shorten their lives; or because they fear that their autonomy will be diminished. Illness is used as a coping mechanism by a relatively small group in most societies. The scope of 'medical illness' depends very much on the contexts condoned by each society. Sexual and psychological problems have been medicalised in Western countries. The problems of poverty and bad housing have been socialised, despite their impact on health: they are thought of as social problems, rather than medical problems.

In semiological terms, there are seven underlying interpretations that describe the reasons for a medical consultation.

1. I have developed a more or less debilitating symptom/sign complex which I think will threaten my duration or quality of life, or my autonomy. I wish you to provide cure or palliation to the best medical standards. (Abdominal pain, temperature, joint pain, sore throat, impotence, depression)

2. I have a symptom/sign which does not affect my activities but whose prognostic significance I fear. I wish you to exercise your skills to confirm or deny what I fear. (Symptomless dark lump on skin, breast lump found during self-examination, symptomless hypertension, raised prostate specific antigen without symptoms)

3. I have neither symptoms nor signs, but I have reason to fear an illness which will shorten or impair my life or restrict my autonomy. I seek reassurance or appropriate management. (Family histories of hepatitis B, colon cancer or Alzheimer's disease, relationship with someone with HIV, hepatitis B or C)

4. I am in good health. I wish you to help me remain that way. (Health maintenance plan, breast screening program)

5. I have evolved or I wish to evolve a pattern of illness as a method of coping with my life. I wish you to reinforce and support this pattern. (Chronic pain syndromes)

6. Someone else has advised me to seek medical help because they perceive that I may have an illness. (Cerebral tumour with personality change, depression, alcoholism, drug dependency)

7. I am suffering from symptoms of existential *angst*, and I do not know where else to turn for help. (Anxiety states, grieving, burnout)

147

These seven consultation types are summarised in Table 10.1, together with a sign representing the presence or absence of a symptom/sign complex, negative impact on quality of life and autonomy and the presence or absence of biomechanical abnormalities.

Table 10.1 Consultation types and their underlying contributing factors

	Symptom/sign complex	Quality of life/ autonomy	Biomechanical abnormalities
Type 1	+	+	+
Type 2	+	−	+
Type 3	−	−	+/−
Type 4	−	−	−
Type 5	+	++	+/−
Type 6	+/−	+/−	+/−
Type 7	++	++	−

The conventional medical response to these implicit positions is largely determined by the content of biomechanical abnormality and the balance between the three components of the presenting problem (the symptom sign complex, quality of life/ autonomy, and biomechanical abnormalities). Many doctors are only comfortable with type 1, 2 and 3 presentations. Many will understand a preoccupation with health maintenance (type 4 presentation), although relatively few are specifically skilled to give advice and design programs. Types 5 to 7 are less easily accommodated within the therapeutic role familiar to most medical graduates, because of the lack of biomechanical content or the disparity between the subjective experience and the objective findings. Psychiatrists handle many of these patients, and other counselling professions and parallel medical practitioners[18] handle most of the rest. The management of such patients, and the place of other practitioners in their management, are not systematically taught in conventional medical curricula, and this is a major gap.

Discourse ethics and the rules of transaction

Medical consultations are clearly directed towards clinical action and, as we saw in chapters 7 and 8, this action should be determined as much by ethics as by science. Habermas[5] evolved a theory of ethics in which the Kantian categorical imperative is replaced by a consensus that must be reached by discourse among those concerned with the effects of an action. Briefly, he proposed two fundamental principles by which he defined his *discourse-ethics*.

> (U) All affected can accept the consequences and the side-effects its general observance can be anticipated to have for the satisfaction of everyone's interests (and these consequences are preferred to those of known alternative possibilities for regulation). This is the universality principle.
>
> (D) Only those norms can claim to be valid that meet (or could meet) with the approval of all affected in their capacity as participants in a practical discourse. This is the principle of practical discourse.

In a sense, a medical consultation can be seen as a discourse-ethics involving at least two people. Other doctors, friends and family members of the patient may also be involved, particularly when mortal questions must be discussed. Habermas used the guidelines of Alexy[19] to describe the rules of the practical discourse involved. Alexy distinguished three levels of action within the process, and suggested that parties to the discourse had to accept certain constraints. In formal terms, Alexy distinguished these levels and their rules in the following way:

I. Logical-semantic level.
   1. No speaker may contradict himself.
   2. Every speaker who applies predicate F to object A must be prepared to apply F to all other objects resembling A in all relevant aspects.
   3. Different speakers may not use the same expression with different meanings.
II. Procedural level.
   1. Every speaker may assert only what he really believes.
   2. A person who disputes a proposition or norm not under discussion must provide a reason for doing so.
III. Process level.
   1. Every subject with the competence to speak and act is allowed to take part in the discourse.
   2. Everyone is allowed to question any assertion whatever.
   3. Everyone is allowed to introduce any assertion whatever.
   4. Everyone is allowed to express his attitudes, desires and needs.
   5. No speaker may be prevented, by internal or external coercion, from exercising his rights as laid down in 1 and 2.

Guidelines of this kind are useful for people who seek a communitarian or negotiated solution to a problem, but are not so appropriate within a medical relationship. Explaining the importance of these 'rules' and allowing medical students to practise using them in clinical encounters, however, may help medical initiates to monitor the progress of communication within the consultative process.

Gadamer used the concept of 'horizons of understanding' in his analyses of discourse as communication.[4] He accepted that people bring different understandings and beliefs to the same problem. The relevance of this concept to medical communication is obvious. The scientific education and preoccupation of doctors may well deviate radically from the lay understanding of patients. In this context, an examination of ideologies[11,12] may be necessary so the two sides in the medical consultation can understand what is being said. The ideologies of herbal medicine and conventional biopositivist medicine are so separated that language may confuse rather than illuminate when someone who believes in herbalism — as many people do in Western countries — needs to consult a conventional practitioner.

Habermas[5] described another potentially divisive difference in values between what he calls the Lifeworld and the System. The Lifeworld stands for the social, cultural and personal domains which depend on communicative action for co-ordination and reproduction. The System — which includes the market and government administration — 'drops out of language', and uses media such as money and power in place of language. The expansion of the System leads to a 'colonisation' of the Lifeworld. This tendency appears in medical relationships because of the intrusions of bureaucracy, law, money and power relationships. Far from helping the doctor–patient relationship, money may interfere with it since that non-language transaction is seen to be so important,[20] and to cut across the immediate need for communication. The ethical problems raised by the accepted need for doctors to make a living were discussed by Rodwin,[21] who wrote: 'Medicine almost inevitably involves a tension between the physicians' commitment to healing others and their economic self-interest.' This tension is often felt by patients and cannot be dismissed lightly, particularly when patients are suffering chronic or terminal illness.

Earlier in this chapter, we noted that the process of taking a medical history and converting it from speech to writing involved a formalising process which took the patient's narrative from the patient's context and placed it in the less personal medical domain. Modern hermeneutic philosophers have examined this textualising process in great detail.

Narrative and text

Ricoeur[6] specified the components of spoken and written communication. 'Narrative' describes multiple forms of story-telling whose common feature is time. Both history and fiction depend on time as the dimension in which they unfold. 'Texts' are units of discourse longer than a sentence, which express the marking, selective and organisational capacities of language. Texts are usually but not necessarily written, and writing represents the ultimate marking function of language. It commits narrative to a form that is further removed from the narrator than speech. Writing makes a text available for criticism and interpretation to other people and at other times. 'Composition' consists of putting a text into the form of a plot (emplotment), selecting and arranging events over time to give a beginning, a middle and end. The plot must be intelligible — each event must contribute to the progress of the story. The ability to follow a story is a sophisticated form of understanding. Taking a medical history implies hearing a clinical narrative, offered by the patient to the doctor, and converting it to a text that is structured, ordered and available for interpretation and understanding by others if necessary.

History as a discipline has become social, political, economic and so on — it is no longer a simple chronicle. A similar trend distorts the medical history, because of the scientific need to remove folk ideology — which may be important to the patient and express fears and beliefs that are central to the experience of illness — from the account of illness. Historians increasingly attempt to emulate the nomological methods of the physical sciences. ('Nomology' means the laws of logical thought.) 'History' reflects the attempted objectivity and analytical stance of the interpreting observer, while 'narrative' reflects the perspective of someone immediately involved and temporally obsessed. The division is never complete, because all history is concerned with time, action and events in the same way as narrative. Any reconstruction of the past calls for imagination. At this point, fiction and history are close: history is coherent narrative conforming to documentation of past events; fiction is coherent narrative that gives meaning to imaginary, but possible, events. A completely objective medical history is therefore impossible.

Both doctor and patient use their differing imaginations in their attempts to make sense of illness according to their different educations, biographies and beliefs.

The illuminating effect of text comes partly from the link between narrative and metaphor, where metaphor is seen as existing at the level of the sentence, rather than the single word. Metaphor makes unlikely attributions to the objects of discussion. A good metaphor expands the understanding of the reader or listener. Metaphor in the medical narrative may be illuminating, but may also risk alienating doctor from patient because it may be dismissed as histrionic or self-indulgent. I once encountered a patient who described her abdominal discomfort as being like 'Toothache without the ache'. This was to me at first an alienating use of words, but reflection reveals its value as an image of preoccupation with a symptom and distress at its effects. Metaphors can be compared to the models of the physical sciences which have the heuristic power to redescribe reality. The countercurrent model of renal tubular function, which compares the tubules of the kidney to an engineering heat exchanger in order to explain its ability to concentrate substances in solution, can be seen as both model and metaphor. Metaphor is not confined to the narrative that the patient offers. Its modelling function has the power to extend the concept of truth, taking it beyond logical coherence or empirical verification. Patients who colour-code their pain or describe the 'suffocation' of their anxiety give insight into the nature of their experience. No metaphor can display its full range outside the context of its text.

Writing down a narrative changes the relationship between author and audience because it becomes and remains available for study by other people at other times. Understanding the text here and now involves understanding yourself confronting the text. This applies to the ordered, written medical history as opposed to the clinical narrative. When my patient complained of abdominal discomfort that resembled toothache without the ache, the effect of the narrative was alienating because the narrative statement seemed meaningless. As text in my notes, available for reflection later and under different circumstances, the statement seemed to make clear the nature of the patient's preoccupation and sense of isolation. Toothache preoccupies the sufferer and makes enjoying ordinary life difficult or impossible. For me to recognise this insight involved extending my understanding of myself, and it is this reflective insight that is at the heart of the hermeneutic experience.

Explanation, understanding and interpretation

Makkreel[22] traced the origins of hermeneutics to Biblical exegesis.[23] Biblical commentators want to define the so-called hermeneutic circle, whereby the whole text can be understood both as a unit and as the sum of its parts, while the parts can be understood as units of structure, but can only be fully understood within the context of their contribution to the whole.

Dilthey,[24] the pioneer of modern secular hermeneutics, distinguished between explanation and understanding. 'Explanation' was the nomological process of the natural sciences, involving prediction from laws and initial conditions. 'Understanding' involved a process of comprehending the parts through an appreciation of the whole. He wrote: 'We explain nature, we understand psychic life.'

Gadamer,[4] in his formulation of a hermeneutic philosophy, pointed out that prejudice — in the literal sense of the word as 'a judgement made in advance of the evidence' — is a vital part of the process of interpretation. Interpreters inevitably hold beliefs and conventions inherited from the past and expressed by the present. Each act of interpretation is irretrievably involved with this synthesis of values, and the romantic notion of hermeneutics as an objective and timeless science of interpretation is not adequate. The prejudices of interpreters are part of the context of a society. Interpreters expand their own horizon of understanding by their work of interpretation. Their success as interpreters depends on their imaginative capacity to find the questions posed by the text or the work of imagination being studied. Understanding is essentially linguistic.

> Language is by no means simply an instrument or tool. For it belongs to the nature of the tool that we master its use, which is to say that we take it in hand and lay it aside when it has done its service. This is not the same as when we take the words of a language, lying ready in the mouth, and with their use let them sink back into the general store of words ... Such an analogy is false because we never find ourselves as consciousness over against the world and, as it were, grasp after a tool of understanding in a wordless condition. Rather, in all our knowledge of ourselves and in all knowledge of the world, we are always encompassed by the language which is our own.[4]

The capacity of some theoretical physicists to think in nonverbal symbols does not change the ordinary dependence on language for communication. Language's complex transparency, its refusal to be pinned down semantically and its capacity to change its meaning with the context, were central features of Wittgenstein's later views.[25] The essence of interpretation, in this perspective, is to say what the author said differently so that it can stay the same. Understanding and explanation work hand in hand in the process of textual interpretation.

'Taking' the history

We can now begin to see what is happening when clinicians 'take' a medical history. They turn the patient's narrative to text, removing the discourse from the patient's lived experience. Doctors assume a set of editorial functions, determined by their need to observe linguistic conventions that may be entirely alien to the patient. What doctors are editing may be the most important manuscript of the patient's life. It is not surprising that many patients with bewildering and unfamiliar symptoms concentrate so much on a narrative chronicle, with obsessive attention to dates. A strict temporality may be immensely important to the patient, because the plot of the narrative has unravelled over a vitally important period of time. This dimension is frequently far less important to doctors, who look for ways to remove the excessive detail that may obscure the bio-mechanical diagnosis, and try to guide the patient as author towards a style that is simple and informative. The doctors' preference for simplification and distancing may cause surprise and disappointment in patients who think that attention to detail is equated with care and accuracy. In their search for understanding, patients may pay minute attention to detail. The way that doctors as interpreters and editors take the history can be seen by patients as a misappropriation of the narrative, not simply as a reasonable appropriation to a text. When taking a complex history, there is an obligation on doctors to explain what they are doing by their editorial condensation, to reassure patients that their grasp of detail is helpful, and that certain aspects of the history may indeed need to be illuminated by that detail. The medical history involves a spectrum of interpretation from the understanding of motives and emotions to the explanation of natural phenomena. We can only understand the 'text' of the medical history through attention to the hermeneutic circle.

Finding a remedy

Most of the time, the potential subtleties of communication do not matter too much. It seems self-evident that common courtesy and common sense will deal with minor problems like the common cold, and yet even such trivial problems may contain deeper ones. Why consult a doctor for a common cold? Most sufferers will treat themselves with a combination of 'folk' and 'medical' therapies. It is probably always wise to run through the checklist of patients' reasons for consulting doctors.

Working within context is a key to interpretation.[6] Words will be interpreted in different contexts of the life histories of patient and doctor and the lived illness of the patient. The education of doctors must include a liberation to 'receive' the history, rather than to 'take' and misappropriate it. The editorial function of doctors in medical consultations involves finding a mutually acceptable form of text by which to objectify as far as possible not only the biomechanical concept of the patient's illness, but also the patient's concept and the values assigned by the patient to the constituents of the experience of illness. The more complex the consultation, the more difficult this will be.

The notion of ideology critique[26] becomes critical in difficult consultations. If the participants cannot define and accept an ideology gap, the discourse between them can never achieve a resolution leading to mutually acceptable action. The Alexy–Habermas guidelines for practical discourse, mentioned above, are likely to break down at all three levels of logic — semantics, procedure and process. When cancer patients seek healing from holistic parallel medicine and yet wish to remain under conventional medical care, there is a need for an uncommon level of understanding between conventional doctors and their patients. Many doctors find it hard to make the leap of understanding required. To understand the other party in this relationship is to challenge one's own self-understanding, to challenge beliefs that are cherished because they make reality out of the confusion of sense-experience and the spiritual crises that are part of the human heritage. Doctors must achieve self-awareness if they achieve anything through the text of the history. Self-awareness brings empathy. Neither greater refinement of medical science nor more precise statements of ethical principles can offer understanding in the same way. If anything can improve communication in the doctor–patient relationship, it will be the kind of insight that springs from understanding, rather than from the scientific explanation that medical graduates are taught to respect above all else. The problems of communication can only be approached by studying and working directly on the processes of communication themselves. There is no short cut.

NOTES

1. Downie RS, Charlton B. The making of a doctor: medical education in theory and practice. Oxford: Oxford University Press, 1992:89–111.
2. Little JM. The problem of the clinical process: a Popperean analysis. Theoretical Surgery 1993; 8:146–50. Also chapter 2 of this book.
3. Toombs SK. The meaning of illness. A phenomenological account of the different perspectives of physician and patient. Dordrecht: Kluwer Academic Publishers, 1992.
4. Gadamer H-G. Philosophical hermeneutics, Linge DE, trans. Berkeley: University of California Press, 1977.
5. Habermas J. Moral consciousness and communicative action, Lenhardt C, Nicholsen SW, trans. Cambridge: Polity Press, 1992.
6. Ricoeur P. From text to action: essays in hermeneutics II, Blamey K, Thompson JB, trans. Evanston, Illinois: Northwestern University Press, 1991.
7. Porter R. The language of quackery in England, 1660–1800. In: Burke P, Porter R, eds. The social history of language. Cambridge: Cambridge University Press, 1987:73–103.
8. 'Quacks' are irregular practitioners of a form of medicine which is based on a system for which there is no accepted support, or on no system at all. Generally, they have no qualifications, unlike practitioners of parallel medicine who have usually graduated from a college or course run by people with similar beliefs.
9. Burke P. Introduction. In: Burke P, Porter R, eds. The social history of language. Cambridge: Cambridge University Press, 1987: 1–20.
10. Wulff HR, Pedersen SA, Rosenberg R. Philosophy of medicine — an introduction, 2nd edn. Oxford: Blackwell Scientific Publications, 1990:172–202.
11. Canguilhem G. Ideology and rationality in the history of the life sciences, Goldhammer G, trans. Cambridge, Massachusetts: MIT Press, 1988.
12. Canguilhem G. The normal and the pathological, Fawcett CR, Cohen RS, trans. New York: Zone Books, 1991:34.
13. Little JM. Quacks, quirks, spells and science. Proceedings of the Medico-Legal Society of New South Wales, 1992; 9:214–23.
14. Cassell EJ. The nature of suffering and the goals of medicine. Oxford: Oxford University Press, 1991.
15. Austin JL. How to do things with words. Oxford: Oxford University Press, 1962.

16. Searle JR. Speech acts: an essay in the philosophy of language. Cambridge: Cambridge University Press, 1969.

17. O'Shea J. Music and medicine: medical profiles of great composers. London: JM Dent, 1993.

18. Parallel medical practitioners are those who practise a form of healing, using theories of health and disease different from those accepted by conventional practitioners. Homoeopathy, chiropractic and herbalism are all guided by perceptions of the body and its functions that are radically different from the perceptions guiding conventional medicine.

19. Alexy R. Eine theorie des praktischen diskurses. In Oelmüler W, ed. Normenbegrüdung. Paderborn: Normendurchsetzung, 1978. Quoted in: Habermas. Moral consciousness and communicative action, Lenhardt C, Nicholsen SW, trans. Cambridge: Polity Press, 1992:87–94.

20. Taylor R. Medicine out of control: the anatomy of a malignant technology. Melbourne: Sun Books, 1979:249–56.

21. Rodwin MA. Medicine, money and morals: physicians' conflicts of interests. Oxford: Oxford University Press, 1993:1.

22. Makkreel RA. Dilthey: philosopher of the human studies. New Jersey: Princeton University Press, 1992.

23. The Barker Bible (or Breeches Bible) of 1599 included profuse hermeneutical marginalia. For example, Genesis 1;12 read: 'And the earth brought forth the bud of the herbe, that seedeth seeds according to his kind, also the tree that beareth fruite, which hath his seed in it selfe according to his kind: and God saw that it was good.' The marginal exegesis explains that this last sentence — 'and God saw that it was good' — 'is so often repeated, to signifie that God made all his creatures to serve to his glory, and to the profite of man: but for sinne they were accursed yet to the elect, by Christ they are restored and serve to their wealth.'

24. Dilthey W. Gessammelte schriften. Quoted in: Makkreel RA. Dilthey: philosopher of the human studies. New Jersey: Princeton University Press, 1992:134.

25. Wittgenstein L. Philosophical investigations. Oxford: Basil Blackwell, 1991.

26. Bleicher J. Contemporary hermeneutics: hermeneutics as method, philosophy and critique. London: Routledge, 1990.

11

Towards a New Medicine

Distressing though the present disillusionment with medicine and its practitioners may be, it is not a new phenomenon.[1] Critiques of medical performance have been formulated since the first written records of medicine, and no doubt there were critiques that antedated writing. Greed, obscurity, arrogance, pomposity, ignorance, coldness — the medical profession has been accused of all these. Great clinicians of the past who were leaders of medical practice, such as Paré, Sydenham, Osler and Blalock, knew perfectly well that good patient management depended on more than medication and good surgical technique. They were scientists, but not necessarily of the reductionist sort. Doctors know that compassion and empathy are qualities that patients admire and seek. But have they the will to improve on the present situation? I have said before that litigation, rising litigation insurance premiums, complaints departments and tighter external controls on medical practice all tell doctors that attitudes and practices need to be changed. But how could this be done?

Only, I think, through education, the curriculum, the establishment of new paradigms for clinicians to follow, and most of all a conscious change from a medical model which is biopositivist to one which is biohumane. Some medical schools are doing what they can. The work of Dr Rita Charon at Columbia University was mentioned. She introduced an undergraduate course[2] which tries to teach an 'empathic stance' rather than the familiar objective and mechanistic one. One exercise involves an interview with a patient suffering a chronic illness. The students must concentrate on the patient's narrative (rather than the medical history) in order to understand how the illness has affected the individual's life. Students then write an account which adopts the patient's voice. Mayo Clinic has introduced a Humanities in Medicine component, in which students confront ethical, moral and communication issues in a Socratic fashion, learning to use empathy as a means of comprehending the dilemmas confronting patients and clinicians. Many other medical schools are doing the same. Downie and Charlton,[3] in their study of medical education, elaborated suggestions for a reduced core curriculum in the pre-clinical years, with student projects that will develop some depth of scientific understanding and a broader involvement in the social sciences. At the same time, they hold that education in the humanities enlarges understanding of the uniqueness of each clinical encounter. 'Whole-person understanding' in the clinical context consists of scientific knowledge of the disease and its physical effects, an understanding of the social impact of the disease, an appreciation of the uniqueness of each clinical history, and an ability to empathise with the particular individual.

Whether these changes will produce a generation of ideal doctors remains to be seen. Students absorb the attitudes of their teachers, and it is difficult to see those attitudes changing in any real way just because the faculty decrees that values must change. Machiavelli[4] pointed out how difficult it is to introduce real change:

> there is nothing more difficult to handle, more doubtful of success, and more dangerous to carry through than initiating changes . . . The innovator makes enemies of all those who prospered under the old order, and only lukewarm support is forthcoming from those

who would prosper under the new. Their support is lukewarm partly from fear of their adversaries, who have the existing laws on their side, and partly because men are generally incredulous, never really trusting new things unless they have tested them by experience.

But there are good reasons to change the present system. Those who seek medical help are saying clearly that they are dissatisfied; and if for some reason doctors distrust the *vox populi*, surely they should listen to those who are telling them most clearly — medical colleagues who have become patients, and are uniquely qualified to tell doctors of the complexities and the failings of the doctor–patient relationship. (This was discussed in chapter 1.) Doctors certainly need to listen: both the public and doctors-as-patients say the same things, and their judgments are far from flattering.

A time for change

Whatever else medical education may be achieving, it does not seem to be educating students in less familiar, non-scientific patterns of thought — in abstract reasoning, in syllogistic thinking, in the principles of *reductio ad absurdum*, in symbolic logic and thought experiments. Yet all these methods have value in trying to teach students something about ethics, and about communication between doctors and patients, between doctors, and between doctors and the wider public. Each can suggest some of the ways to enhance communication. I want the the distinction between science and the humanities to be abandoned, as much in the medical curriculum as in civilisation at large. Karl Popper[5] said: 'Labouring the difference between science and the humanities has long been a fashion and has become a bore.' It is more than a bore. It is profoundly destructive. In medical teaching, it is possible to link science and humane practice by using the science to deal with ethical, legal and existential, value-laden problems as they would arise in problem-based teaching episodes. An example of a learning package of this kind appears in the appendix to this book.

It is an article of faith that there is a nexus between healing, communication and the humanities. Osler was sure that reading made a better person and a better person made a better doctor. In his essay *Books and Men*,[6] he wrote: 'This high education so much needed today is not given in the school, is not to be bought in the market place, but is to be wrought out in each of us for himself; it is the silent influence of character on character.' Osler considered that reading great writers was part of medical education because it was part of being a "gentleman". Aldridge,[7] took the argument further in a modern context, postulating that aesthetics could be a vital part of clinical communication. He wrote: 'In artistic expression we have the possibility of making perceptible an inner experience . . . In this way we can ask of our research that it expresses what it is to be human, what it is to be well and what it is to fall sick.'

Olafson,[8] in a thoughtful examination of the problems faced by contemporary literary studies, has followed Gadamer in his argument for the continuing importance of hermeneutics. He said that what matters in approaching a literary text is

> the idea that what we encounter in a work is a truth-claim that we ourselves must confront if we are to 'understand' that work itself. In so doing, at least in favorable circumstances, we effect a rapprochement between the vision implicit in the work and our own prior beliefs and through our acknowledgment (or perhaps one should say 'our negotiation') of the truth-claim it makes, it acquires a bearing on our lives. Examples of such application are not at all hard to find as any thoughtful reader of Oedipus Rex or Don Quixote will surely agree.

These understandings of the literary text have much in common with the understandings of the medical history, discussed in chapter 10.

The case of medicine

The distressed and ill seek comfort and relief wherever they can. Medicine in all its forms has provided — and still provides — the best care for a range of ills, and it has done so by concentrating on a direct and personal relationship between patient and doctor. Medicine's success in dealing with diseases that rob people of life and quality of life has been achieved at enormous cost. No matter which system of delivery a country uses, a significant proportion of its GDP is spent on health. Furthermore, science and technology have begun to replace personal rapport and physical contact in the diagnostic and therapeutic processes, and there are jobs and money in science and technology. This appeals to economically rational people, and has caused an alliance between scientists, technocrats, businesspeople and transnational companies. Medicine is big business, and politically important. It no longer belongs to doctors and their patients, but to policy makers and investors.

Professor Anne Sefton has shown that literature and language skills predict 'success' in the medical undergraduate course at the University of Sydney far better than the mathematics and science skills which earn the students entry to the medical faculty. This is scarcely surprising, since communication is still necessary to both sides in medical transactions. Selecting medical undergraduates more on the basis of language skills might lead to a generation of clinicians once more alert to the simple meanings of the complex language of pain, fear and loss. Good communicators are both expressive and receptive, and often choose to express and receive art, music and literature, as well as the often coded messages of patients. But compulsory literary or art appreciation or creative writing courses will not create a sensitive generation, any more than a compulsory course in comparative religion would produce a generation of theologists. It is necessary to accept that there are some who will always be indifferent to aesthetics, and yet be competent physicians.

Compulsory creativity?

All creativity attempts to set out a realisation and to test and share the validity of the insight. Not everyone can paint, compose music or write poetry, but everyone can look at, listen to and read the products of gifted people. In these ways anyone with motivation can experience the creative act and grapple with the problems of creativity. The very process of struggling creatively with problems, whether in literature or science, may be the most important single experience for humanists in medicine. In chapter 2, I quoted Popper:[5]

> I also suggest that the much discussed problem of the transference of learning from one discipline to another is closely connected with gaining experience in wrestling with live problems. Those who have learned only to apply some theoretical framework to the solving of problems . . . cannot expect that their training will help them much in another specialism. It is different for those who have themselves wrestled with problems, especially if their understanding, clarification, and formulation, proved difficult.

The preoccupations of literature are the preoccupations of patients and doctors — love and birth and death, pain and loss and suffering, grief, anger, elation and tranquillity, balance and harmony and rhythm. Doctors in their literary writing may give a truer idea of the tensions of their profession than popular literature and television. Chekhov was a doctor, and the vague and dithering physicians of his plays are at once wise and foolish, trite in the face of everyday complaints, yet wise with experience in the face of death and loss.

As Aldridge[7] suggested, patients in their writing, their painting and their music can share with doctors the unexpressed agony of the soul that may be a part of the medical experience. Sensitive writers can express the anger of bereavement, the puzzlement of the spectator at the bedside. Stories and poems have their own 'truth content'. When Dylan Thomas, helplessly mourning his dying father, wrote:[9]

> And you my father, there on the sad height,
> Curse, bless, me now with your fierce tears, I pray.
> Do not go gentle into that good night.
> Rage, rage against the dying of the light,

he showed the anger and pain of watching death with more immediacy than any lecture on the subject.

Downie and Charlton[3] pointed out that science is concerned with generalisations and laws, and encourages medical students to see individual patients as members of groups. The uniqueness of individuals and their quest for autonomy are best understood through the humanities, because poets, novelists, playwrights, painters and sculptors all deal with individuals. Doctors, patients and the community should benefit from these insights. But bureaucrats, politicians, investors and many doctors will remain impervious, unless humanists can learn to measure and communicate the benefits to be gained from the humanist view of healing — to place them in Popper's world 3,[5] the world of objective knowledge and thought, where concepts can be discussed and criticised, where theories live or die.

Humanism and the practice of persuasion

Humanism is concerned with persuasion. Its communication is rhetoric. This is not wrong, nor is it a criticism of the communication system of humanism, but it is important to acknowledge the potential problem. Novelists and poets persuade by overpowering reductionist scientific logic with another dimension of pluralist logic, and we respond with a feeling of truth identified and made manifest. This skill in persuasion is part of humanist communication, and it uses a logic different from that of science. There may be no scientific proof of what is said or revealed, but the revelation is no less 'true'. It expresses the truth which resides in ethics, morality and aesthetics.

Medicine must accept external controls, because of its economic and political importance. These externals only become intolerable when they dominate the practice of medicine and interfere with doctors' capacity to deliver their complex services in a simple and direct relationship. To counter the arguments of bureaucrats and economists, doctors must have sound counter-arguments. Information from controlled trials to support medical treatment is available for only about 15% of interventions, a figure derived by the Congressional Office of Technology Assessment.[10] We have already seen that only about 1% of medical publications represent 'good' science. Disinformation from advertising, vested interests and poor science is available, however, to support almost anything. Eddy[10] from Duke University and the Marburg group of Lorenz[11] showed that good science can be handled in ways that make powerful sense to clinicians and convincing arguments to administrators. Some of these techniques were mentioned earlier. If doctors are to retain their role as medical practitioners and philosophers of healing, they must realise that their new humanity will only be realised by an alliance with the new scientists of decision and social planning. They must also accept that the 'new' humanism includes this science. There is nothing really new in that message. Greek and Roman humanists, Renaissance artists and Victorian reformers all knew that science was a part of humanism.

Chapter 1 noted that there is biological and epidemiological evidence that death is inevitable, that cellular systems have a life of about 90 years,[12,13] and that the mean duration of life has increased by about 26 years in this century. This phase of achievement belongs to the 20th century, and if health is to be judged by mean duration of life, medicine has reached the phase of diminishing returns. Increasingly, the contemporary achievement is, and must continue to be, an improvement in the quality of life. Social scientists and clinicians in many countries are struggling to define and measure quality of life, and to incorporate the measures into a new clinical science. Traditional humanists must not dismiss these efforts as attempts to define the undefinable. Anything which can be communicated can also be measured, and the humanist concerns are communication and quality of life. These new scientists are part of the humanist movement, and the humanists must join them in order to lead and to follow.

'Good data', science and politics

The uneasiness in the current stand-off between the alliance of scientists and politicians on one side and the humanists in medicine on the other is easy enough to define. It is the tension between collectivism and individualism. Although scientists and politicians may not think of themselves as having a common cause, both groups are concerned with 'good data', with statistics and mass effects, with uniformity and best practice. The scientists, who should be the allies of the clinical practitioners, are persuaded by the politicians and the fund providers to make a common cause, based around large numbers, probabilities, utilities and statistical benefit, and ultimately the laudable desire to secure value for money. But medicine — as opposed to public health — has always dealt with individual well-being. The confusion between medicine and health is a serious matter, and it afflicts both politicians and medical profession. Medicine is the process of healing the individual; health is the political and social expression of medicine. Both are ethically 'good', and both ultimately concern themselves with individual health and well-being. By convention, medical education attempts to prepare its students to practise both disciplines. Commonly, however, medical courses fail to make clear the interdependence of the two — the requirement of clinicians for statistics and probabilities, and the need of health experts to understand the nature of illness and individual suffering and disability.

From $n = \propto$ back to $n = 1$

Politicians and scientists like to think in terms of large numbers, where n is equal to hundreds or thousands or preferably hundreds of thousands. For scientists, large numbers mean greater statistical validity and smaller confidence intervals. For politicians, large groups made uniform by mathematics are better economic and voting units to consider than fragmented, more angular and less definable ones. For clinicians in daily practice, $n = 1$ at every consultation. Each person remains unique, no matter how well he or she conforms to group descriptors. Each consultation is a unique transaction, in which advice may be given and accepted, rejected or modified. For an individual patient, there may not be a 'best' treatment, to be prescribed by a clinician or a bureaucrat. The 'best' choice may depend on patient preferences and available resources. Finding that 'best' choice is the joint task of clinician and patient, and that is the stage when communication and the humanist skills of judgment are pre-eminent, when heuristics replace statistics and intuition replaces science.

Clinicians need not lose their devotion to their $n = 1$ relationship with each patient. An earlier chapter mentioned the oncologist Freireich[14] from the MD Anderson Hospital commenting that when doctors and statisticians become ill, they ask 'Who is the best doctor for this problem?' not 'Which multi-centre controlled trial would be best for me?' Clinicians must remain grateful for the information that scientists and bureaucrats can generate, and must encourage them to gather, summarise and disseminate knowledge so that communications with individual patients will be better informed and clearer. Clinicians must also ask politicians to define and declare their policies towards both health and medicine and the rationales that underpin these policies, so that clinicians and their patients can understand better the supply-side economics of medicine.

Clinicians should not, however, allow themselves to be forced into the morally untenable position of being both the suppliers and the rationers of services. The disposition of money within the national budget is a political decision. If services are to be limited or modified because of budgetary constraints, there is a clear political responsibility. This is not judgmental. Ethically, a decision to limit the health budget may be good, bad or neutral, depending on the alternative use to which the money is put. What matters is the political nature of the decision. As we saw in chapter 1, the medical profession can offer services and the public can demand services. There would be no end to the expenses generated if these forces were allowed free rein. The guidelines that define limitations must be developed, with help from clinicians, and publicised. Once they are defined, both clinicians and patients can understand the limitations to availability of services.

To summarise, humanism and the humanities have the potential to open the way to better understanding and communication, to a better professional and political performance and a better image of the profession in the eyes of its real public. They also offer medical graduates a richer life, a greater understanding of their own achievements, a protection against isolation, a sense of place and another sense of purpose. They help to augment the practical wisdom required for and generated by the one-to-one relationship that is the basis of medical practice. Olafson[8] wrote 'that literature, unlike endocrinology or plasma physics, addresses us in our capacity as human beings, and . . . this entails a different constituency and a different set of priorities . . . from those that are appropriate for scientific disciplines'. The humanities offer an experience of the world of feelings and values, which can be as profound as people allow it to be. They should be a part of medical education.

NOTES

1. Much of the material in this chapter was deleivered as an oration for the Humanities in Medicine Committee of Mayo Clinic, and was published as Communication and the humanities: the nature of the nexus. Mayo Clinic Proceedings 1993; 68:921–4.
2. Charon R. Doctor-patient/reader-writer: learning to find the text. Soundings 1989; 72:137–52.
3. Downie RS, Charlton B. The making of a doctor: medical edu-

cation in theory and practice. Oxford: Oxford University Press, 1992.

4. Machiavelli N di B. New principalities acquired by one's own arms and prowess, in: Bull G, trans. The prince. Harmondsworth: Penguin, 1983:51.

5. Popper KR. Objective knowledge: an evolutionary approach. Oxford: Clarendon Press, 1979.

6. Osler W. Books and men, In: Aequinimitas with other addresses to medical students, nurses and practitioners of medicine. London: HK Lewis & Co. 1948.

7. Aldridge D. Aesthetics and the individual in the practice of medical research. Discussion paper. Journal of the Royal Society of Medicine 1991; 84:147–50.

8. Olafson FA. 'Human sciences' or 'humanities': the case of literature. In: French PA, Uehling TE Jr, Wettstein HK, eds. Midwest studies in philosophy vol xv: the philosophy of the human sciences. Notre Dame, Indiana: University of Notre Dame Press, 1990:183–93.

9. Thomas D. Do not go gentle into that good night. In: Collected poems 1934–52. London: JM Dent, 1974.

10. Eddy DM. Medicine, money, and mathematics. American College of Surgeons Bulletin 1992; 77:36–49.

11. Lorenz W. Current status of theoretical surgery: marginal example or model for systematic medical decision-making? Theoretical Surgery 1992; 7:135–6.

12. Hayflick L. The cell biology of human aging. Scientific American 1980; 242:42–9.

13. Fries JF. Aging, natural death and the compression of morbidity. New England Journal of Medicine 1980; 303:130–5.

13. For heuristic, see Glossary.

14. Freireich EJ. The randomized clinical trial as an obstacle to clinical research. In: Delaney JP, Varco RL, eds. Controversies in surgery II. Philadelphia: WB Saunders, 1983:5–12.

12

A Summary

I would like to conclude by summarising the argument set out in this book, and by anticipating some of the implications of the call for reform that it makes.

1. Medicine starts with and continues to be justified by a tacit belief in the primacy of the human species. If this were not so, there would be no problem, since health and individual healing would have no more value than, say, veterinary medicine or botany. Because we believe that the human condition and the human capacity for suffering are special, however, we vote a large fraction of the country's wealth and income to health and medicine. We believe that it is worthwhile to invest in this way because we accept that a developed society should protect and improve the health of its citizens. This devotion to the health and well-being of individuals is common to clinicians and specialists in public health. Clinicians treat sick individuals, and contribute to the well-being of society, while specialists in public health promote individual health and well-being by improving the health of the population. Without an acceptance that the health of individuals is important, neither could comfortably justify their existence.

2. It is this *a priori* assumption that justifies both the science and the ethics of medicine. The science is designed to elucidate in a reductionist fashion the mechanisms of disease. Medical scientists implicitly assume that explanation must precede cure, and that elucidating the basic mechanisms is a necessary start to preventing or reversing disease. *Reductionist science has become the most important element of progress within the present biomechanical model of human health and disease.* But it is not enough to justify medicine as a specialism on its own. Without an ethical base, reductionist science can become corrupt, as shown by the Nazi experiments during the Second World War, or the Willowbrook trial.

   a. The ethical and bioethical movements have evolved particularly since the Second World War because the development of medical science needed to be related to the rights of the ill, and because the principle of autonomy was seen as central to the preservation of those rights. The principles of beneficence, non-maleficence, autonomy, justice and professional behaviour probably do more to define the medical profession's existence than anything else. Many scientists do biological work in laboratories, but only the medical profession is entrusted to apply science to individual humans because it is assumed to subscribe to an ethical code which will protect each person's welfare.

3. It is this unique ethical responsibility for human distress that makes specialised communication so important. Empathic, fluent and intelligible communication with patients should be one of the main goals of a medical curriculum. The skills required to communicate with politicians, bureaucrats and the media will be required by relatively few people, but the principles needed for public communication should be known by all.

4. Specialised communication requires a special dimension of understanding to overcome the specific problems which arise at the interface between professional and folk knowledge.

The lay appreciation of many words, such as cancer, shock, system, stroke and heart attack, is quite different from the professional understanding. There are emotional overtones to many words, and using them in explanations may convey messages of death and suffering which the doctor has long forgotten. Present medical courses concentrate on a positivist precision in language, and discourage sympathy for the language usages of the average man-in-the-street.

5. There are formidable barriers to successful communication across the divide between doctors and patients. There are clear signs that medicine has lost much of its standing. Government control, hostile media, complaints departments and increasing litigation warn that the communication barriers are harming the standing of the medical profession, and threatening to limit the very real good that it has the power to do.

6. Some of these barriers can be identified, and they include:
   a. The 'Kuhnian gap'. Kuhn[1] pointed out that as a science becomes more 'successful', it becomes harder to communicate the latest advances. Eventually, scientists are able only to communicate with other scientists working within the same discipline. This difficulty has been well demonstrated by quantum mechanics and by cosmological concepts like string theory or singularities.
   b. The difficulty of explaining probability. Most medical science, particularly clinical science, produces data that is essentially probabilistic. It is not, like the physical sciences, deterministic. The lay public, however, read and watch the miracles of physical science through the interpretations of the media and form the impression that all 'good' science is deterministic, and that medicine is a science. The profession does little to contradict this view, and is indeed firmly attached to the notion of science as the way to the future of medicine. It is therefore difficult for doctors to express and for patients to understand that medical advice about the outcome of treatment is nearly always indefi-

nite, because it can only be expressed as a probability, without any guarantee that an individual patient will be one of those who will obtain a desired (or undesirable) outcome.

c. Information flood. Medical information is generated at the staggering rate of 34 000 articles each month in medical journals.[2] Doctors cannot be fully informed about the whole field of medicine, nor even about their own specialty. Patients have still less chance of being able to appreciate the knowledge and information that refers to their specific problems. Neither doctors nor patients are usually skilled at separating information from knowledge, and many are unaware of the division.

d. The media likewise often promote disinformation by hailing some interesting scientific development as a 'breakthrough'. Other groups with vested interests may do the same, claiming results for drugs or operations that have not been adequately tested. This tendency can be seen in the present wave of enthusiasm for laparoscopic surgery.

e. The politicisation of medicine adds to the difficulties of communication. Rival parties denigrate each other's health policies, and promise to address the shortcomings which they feel are important — or can be made to seem important — in the minds of voters. Medical practitioners also tend to adopt political stances, and to adhere to them when wisdom and judgment might recommend a non-partisan approach.

f. There are other vested interests in and around medicine. There are special interest groups representing patients (devoted to child health, women's issues, cancer and heart disease, as examples) or representing specialties within medicine (orthopaedic surgery, general practitioners, emergency room doctors and many others) which may distort the public perceptions of such important issues as allocation of resources.

g. Public expectations are generated by cultural commitments, the level of prosperity, education, political theory
and practice, the media and the folk inheritance of each
subculture. Once formed, expectations are difficult to
change, particularly when it is necessary to lower them. A
culture of science and materialism creates expectations
that the power of science can solve any problem.

h. This leads to a confusion of wants and needs. Society
largely endorses the notion of health as a right. The acceptance of this right is linked to a belief that all services
should be available to all members of society, and that
everyone should have access to a science that saves and
prolongs life indefinitely. The expectation that medical
science should cure every illness is translated into cure as a
basic right.

i. Medicine unwittingly encourages these expectations by
emphasising science more than humane understanding.
The image that medicine adopts for itself is one of the
scientist-technician, whose clinical gaze sees the mechanical defects of the sick body, and whose technical and
technological skills can service and repair what is wrong.
The empirical, positivist element in medicine has overwhelmed the humane, devaluing discourse and rendering
language less important than objective measurements and
structural appearances. The reward and granting systems
within medicine continue to signal that positivism is good,
and that value-laden endeavour is worthy but ultimately
suspect. The human genome project will attract more support than any research and practice in palliative care.

j. The problem of curing for profit. The motives of most
doctors are ultimately good, but the necessity for payment
creates problems. It does not matter much whether individuals pay doctors directly or through tax: payment
occurs, and the fact of payment professionalises the transaction and creates a further set of vested interests. Doctors

want to preserve or increase their income, government wants to minimise the cost of the health budget, patients want to shift responsibility for health. Like it or not, the medical profession is often regarded as greedy. The market element in medicine may even actively interfere with the language of communication that should be available to both doctors and patient.[3]

7. If these matters are to be taken seriously, very profound changes will be required of medical practitioners. Although it must help to be made aware of the problems, awareness will not necessarily translate into a reform of action and practice. *It is unlikely that re-education of the present members of the profession would succeed in producing real change.* Radical change is more likely to occur if the education of medical undergraduates is reformed.

   a. Re-educating the present profession. There are forces within the medical profession that will resist change. Although it will be possible to explain why curricular reform is desirable, most senior members of the clinical profession will be reluctant to endorse and help to implement radical change, for the following reasons.

      i. Most are in well-established clinical and academic practices, which are successful and providing a familiar clinical and research environment. There is therefore little incentive to change.

      ii. Those who do much of the teaching, particularly in the clinical years, were taught a different way. They teach comfortably in that same way, and often teach very well. There is little motivation to learn a new methodology of problem-based learning, particularly as this unfamiliar technique will take more time than the traditional pedagogical methods.

      iii. Clinical practitioners have their own programs of continuing education and re-certification. These programs concentrate on clinical practice, not on undergraduate teaching methods, and require a significant time commitment. Asking these clinical teachers to spend even more time on learning undergraduate teaching methods is unreasonable.

b. Educating the next generation of medical graduates thus emerges as the only way in which the profession may achieve major change. The principles that underlie change of this magnitude will include the following.

   i. Selection of older students with undergraduate training in many fields, and with proven ability to think conceptually and to use language effectively.

   ii. A change in teaching direction, rather than content, toward problem-based learning in the clinical component, while preserving the scientific content of the basic teaching of form and function.

   iii. Teaching by precept, example, assessment and reward the importance of communications, ethics, information handling, critical assessment and continuing education.

8. New teaching methods must be evaluated. If radical reform is initiated, the medical faculties must spend time, money and effort to determine what happens to medical students during and long after their medical course.

NOTES

1. Kuhn TS. The structure of scientific revolutions, 2nd edn. Chicago, Illinois: University of Chicago Press, 1970.
2. Arndt KA. Information excess in medicine: overview, relevance to dermatology, and strategies for coping. Archives of Dermatology 1992; 128:1249–56.
3. Brand A. The force of reason: an introduction to Habermas' theory of communicative action. Sydney: Allen & Unwin, 1990.

Glossary

A priori A *priori* knowledge is held independent of experience. The term is also applied to arguments that reach conclusions based on *a priori* knowledge.

Bayes' theorem An expression which modifies the initial (prior) probability of an occurrence in the light of new data. In medicine, Bayes' theorem is typically applied to diagnostic test results. In its most familiar form, it has the following formula:

$$P(D|S) = \frac{P(S|D)P(D)}{P(S|D)P(D) + P(S|\bar{D})P(\bar{D})}$$

where $P(D|S)$ is the probability of the disease being present when a particular test is positive (the true positive rate), $P(S|D)$ is the probability of the test being positive when the disease is known to be present, $P(D)$ is the prevalence or probability of the disease in the relevant population, $P(S|\bar{D})$ the probability that the test result will be positive in the absence of the disease (false positive rate), and $P(\bar{D})$ is the probability that the disease will not be present in the same community.

Biohumane The term used in this book to describe a model of medicine which recognises the real importance of the subjective and value-laden aspects of the experience of health and illness, while continuing to emphasise the importance of scientific medicine.

Biopositivism The prevailing intellectual model in medicine throughout the 20th century. It conceives disease to be a set of definable abnormalities of structure and function, which can be objectively (scientifically and empirically) demonstrated and measured. It tends to be realist, materialist and reductionist in orientation. Disorders of function, such as irritable gut syndrome, pose problems for biopositivism until structural disorders at any level of the reductionist schema can be identified. The human genome project represents the extreme expression of the orientation and beliefs of the biopositivist ideology. It is also known as biomechanicalism, biophysicalism and biomedicalism.

Constructivism A view of science which holds that the subject matter of research depends on the theoretical assumptions of the scientific community and therefore does not exist as something real and independent of the beliefs and theoretical commitments of scientists.

Covering law model An account of scientific explanation which holds that valid explanation consists of inference from a law of nature, together with a statement of initial or boundary conditions.

Deduction The process of reaching valid conclusions from premises: 'All men are mortal. Socrates is a man. Therefore, Socrates is mortal.' If the premises are true, so is the conclusion.

Deductive–nomological explanation An explanation by inference under the covering law model. Often considered to be the most powerful explanatory model. 'Cutaneous sensation is conveyed by intact peripheral nerves. This peripheral nerve has been cut. Therefore, there is no cutaneous sensation in the distribution of this nerve.'

Deontology The science of duty or moral obligations.

Determinism The view, stated strongly by Laplace among others, that the final state of a system is determined by its initial state. In particle science, determinism has been challenged by quantum mechanics, which has reduced small-scale systems involving fundamental particles to probabilities. Heisenberg's uncertainty principle states that it is impossible to measure the position and momentum of a fundamental particle, such as an electron, simultaneously with any accuracy. Thus statements about the position and velocity of a particle can only be given as statistical probabilities, rather than determinate certainties.

Dialectic In the Socratic sense, dialectic is the conversational or discursive method of examining and challenging a person's views. In Plato's sense, it has come to describe the supreme knowledge which 'gives an account' of everything. Hegel extended the meaning of the term to cover what he held to be the logical path that all thought must follow — that is, a process of contradiction and reconciliation.

Diethylstilboestrol A synthetic female sex hormone first synthesised in 1938. At different times, it was used to treat menopausal symptoms, acne, some types of cancer, control of growth in adolescent girls, and recurrent miscarriage and to suppress lactation. In the 1970s, it was realised that its use was associated with vaginal sarcoma in the children of treated mothers, and probably with breast cancer in women who took the drug.

DRGs (diagnosis related groupings) A device for assessing medical practice against relevant norms. Each diagnosis is assigned a normal hospital stay and a cost weight. Profiles of practice can then be assessed against established performance, and funds allocated accordingly.

Empiricism The view that knowledge can only be based on sensory experience. The British philosophers (Hobbes, Locke and Hume, among many others) elaborated empiricism at the expense of idealism.

Epidemiology The study of the incidence and transmission of disease in populations, especially with the aim of controlling it.

Epistemology The philosophical study of the nature, origins and limitations of knowledge.

181

Falsificationism Karl Popper claimed that a theory or hypothesis was 'scientific' if and only if criteria could be defined which could refute its claims. Thus, the claim that the moon is made of green cheese is a scientific claim, because it can conceivably be falsified. The claim that piety is better than altruism, on the other hand, cannot be falsified, and is therefore not scientific.

Gestalt shift Thomas Kuhn considered that science progresses episodically, rather than smoothly. During stable periods of normal science, scientists work within the prevailing paradigms, solving puzzles generated by the paradigms. As more and more questions go unanswered by the prevailing paradigms, science becomes unstable, until a revolution occurs and the paradigms change quickly by the process of gestalt shift. *Gestalt* is a German word meaning the holistic configuration or organisation of the whole, which is more than the constituent parts.

Hermeneutics Originally, the study of interpretation of texts, more specifically Biblical texts. The term has been extended to cover inquiry into the understanding of human behaviour, speech and institutions generally. Existentialists also used the term to cover inquiry into the meaning of human existence.

Heuristic The adjective means 'concerned with ways of solving problems or of finding out things'. The noun refers to incremental problem-solving aimed at reaching an unknown solution by following a pathway such as a decision algorithm.

Hodgkin's disease A variety of lymph gland cancer which is often curable by modern chemotherapy and radiotherapy.

Holism Basically, the view that the totality of entities and systems is more than the simple sum of their parts. There are ontological, semantic and epistemological views of holism.

Hypothesis A scientific claim that has been advanced for examination, before there is evidence to accept it or reject it.

Hypothetico–deductive method An account of theory testing whereby predictions are made on the basis of the theory, together with statements of auxiliary or limiting conditions. The accuracy of the predictions is then tested.

Induction The process of reaching a general conclusion on the basis of repeated observations: 'All humans so far observed have died; therefore all humans will die.'

Inference Drawing a conclusion from a set of premises. The process of reaching a conclusion may be deductive or inductive.

Law A causal or statistical relationship between two or more elements: $F = ma$, for example. Laws allow predictions and postulation about what will happen if certain initial conditions are met.

Lithotripsy A method of smashing stones, usually in the kidneys or gall bladder, using instruments or shock waves. The stones can then be passed naturally.

Logical positivism or *logical empiricism* A school of philosophers of science who held that verification was the essential feature defining science. Their views were strongly opposed by Popper, who held that potential falsification was the essential demarcation.

Materialism A view that all phenomena can be explained in mechanical terms.

Metaphysics The fundamental study of reality. Logical positivists dismissed metaphysical inquiry as meaningless because it could not be subjected to objective verification.

Naturalism A view that the methods of the natural sciences can be used in all areas of inquiry, and that all phenomena are governed by natural laws.

Nomology The science of laws, more particularly in modern use the science of the laws of the mind or laws of logical thought.

Nosology The system of classifying diseases.

Objectivity The property of a theory or hypothesis or a method of investigation that reflects phenomena as independent of the beliefs of the observer.

Ontology The branch of metaphysics concerned with the nature of existence. Also, the system of entities postulated by a theory.

Paradigm A term used by Thomas Kuhn to describe the set of core theories and beliefs that determine the methods and interpretation of scientific inquiry. In a more general sense, it refers to a way of viewing things by way of accepted assumptions and clear models. The geocentric model of Ptolemaic astronomy was the accepted paradigm in astronomy, until it was replaced by the heliocentric model, which then became the paradigm for a later era.

Positivism A philosophical belief in the primacy of 'positive facts' as the only knowable matters. In this view, speculation about cause, origins or purposes is pointless. *See also* biopositivism.

Probability In its frequental sense, probability expresses numerically the likelihood of an event or observation. In its subjective sense, it reflects the strength of belief in a theory or hypothesis.

Rationalism The term used by philosophers to describe the view that knowledge is intrinsic to the reasoning process, and must therefore begin from an *a priori* base. For example, Descartes' famous 'Cogito, ergo sum' ('I think, therefore I am') as the starting point for a philosophy based on reasoning from an *a priori* assumption.

Realism The view that phenomena dealt with by a theory exist independently of the minds that examine them.

Reductionism Understanding complex theories, concepts and systems in terms of simpler concepts or their isolated components.

Relativism The view of epistemology which holds that what is 'known' is determined by the beliefs of a particular community at a particular time. According to relativists, there are no grounds for believing in absolute and immutable truths.

Sarcoma A sarcoma is a cancer of connecting or supporting tissues, such as muscle or fibrous tissue, rather than of the lining tissues or the glands which are involved in the commoner types of cancer, such as those of the bowel, prostate or breast.

Scientific realism The belief that the objects of scientific study exist independently of the minds that study them.

Semantic The meaning of words and other linguistic forms.

Stochastic A word describing a process which is not deterministic. The initial state of a system does not determine the final state. It only defines the probabilities of alternative final states.

Structuralism A view which maintains that social and linguistic systems are not well analysed by the methods of the natural sciences, and that they are best understood by examining structural relationships between the components of the language or social system.

Subjectivity The property of a theory or hypothesis that reflects the personal aspects of an individual, rather than those of an independently existing world.

Syllogism An argument with two premises and a conclusion.

Teleology A theory which holds that anything can only be understood by considering the ends toward which it is directed.

Theory Any general and systematic account, usually expressed in abstract terms, and sometimes making use of unobservable entities to provide explanations.

Trope A figure of speech, such as a metaphor, in which the words are used in another sense than the literal one.

Truth The OED defines truth as 'Conformity with fact; agreement with reality', but for the modern philosopher there is no such easy answer. The OED definition encapsulates the correspondence theory, in which truth is simply that which corresponds to the observed facts. The coherence view is holistic, and insists that a statement is true if and only if it coheres with other statements held to be true. The redundancy theory holds that truth is expressed if and only if the statement that 'X is true' can be restated without using the term 'is true'. Thus, the statement that 'It is true that untreated cardiac arrest is fatal' can be restated as 'Untreated cardiac arrest is fatal' and such a statement is true. The concept of truth is one where intuitive notions prove to be inadequate when they are examined systematically.

APPENDIX

A Humane Medicine
Teaching Package

In this appendix I wish to set out a teaching package which incorporates some of the ideas examined in this book. It represents a learning episode for medical students, in which an incurable condition (carcinoma of the gall bladder) is used as a reference point. The students work out the diagnostic approach, and are then challenged to use their science-based knowledge to deal with ethical and hermeneutic problems.

I recognise that this material will only have meaning for those with medical knowledge, and I have therefore used medical terminology and some abbreviations without explanation.

Resource material

1. Reading list
   Blumgart LH, ed. Surgery of the liver and biliary tract. Edinburgh: Churchill Livingstone, 1988:791–896.
   Treatment of pain in patients with cancer of the pancreas or bile ducts. Preece PE, Cuschieri A, Rosin RD, eds. In: Cancer of the bile ducts and pancreas. Philadelphia: WB Saunders, 1989: 291–312.
   Way LW, ed. Current surgical diagnosis and treatment. Appleton & Lange, 1991:550–2, 1207–46.

2. Patient/surrogate
3. Electrolytes/urea/creatinine (EUC), liver function tests (LFTs), full blood count (FBC) and coagulation screen for patient with upper gastrointestinal carcinoma
4. Computerised tomogram (CT) showing large carcinoma of the gall bladder with liver metastases. Abdominal ultrasound (US) of same patient
5. Unobstructed endoscopic retrograde cholangiopancreatogram (ERCP)
6. Teaching participants
   a. Pathologist
   b. Physician/surgeon
   c. Oncologist
   d. Pain management team
   e. Palliative care team
   f. Counselling specialist

Teaching methodology

The teaching method is problem-oriented. The case vignette, appropriate investigations and reading list will be available to students before the session. Student discussion is guided by mentor, using details of desired knowledge. Evaluation of the session is completed by using the checklist of items at the end of this package.

Résumé

A 58-year-old man presents to you, accompanied by his wife. For three months, he has experienced increasing pain in the right upper quadrant of the abdomen. The pain now goes through to his back on the right side. The pain is dull, constant and wakes him regularly in the early hours of the morning. It is partly relieved by paracetamol. His appetite has progressively worsened, and he has lost 8 kg in weight since the pain began. He has noticed no pruritus. His urine has not been dark, nor his stools pale. He has been a little constipated. He has experienced increasing nausea, but no vomiting. He feels constantly fatigued, and is now unable to work at his well-paid job as an accountant in a small firm. He drinks alcohol socially about once each week, and he does not smoke. His general health has been good, and he is taking no medications apart from paracetamol. His father died of liver cancer, and he thinks that he may have the same condition.

On examination, he has clearly lost weight. He looks unwell. His conjunctivae are pale and the palmar creases have lost their colour. There is a 6 cm by 4 cm mass in the right upper quadrant which is hard and slightly tender. It moves with respiration, and can best be felt just lateral to the border of the rectus abdominis muscle. The liver edge can be felt 3 cm below the right costal margin lateral to the mass, and it is firm, smooth and not tender. The mass appears to be in or on the liver. There are no other masses in the abdomen. The spleen is not enlarged and there is no ascites. There is no lymphadenopathy. There are no stigmata of chronic liver disease. He is not jaundiced.

Phase 1: First impressions and proposed next moves

1. What diagnoses come to mind?
2. Is the condition likely to be benign or malignant?
3. Is there any possible significance to the family history?
4. What investigation regime might secure the quickest diagnosis and the quickest profile of the patient? Justify each of the tests and explain what use you might make of abnormal results that you may get from your tests.

Checklist

- FBC EUC LFTs
- Hepatitis serology
- Iron studies
- Tumour markers
- Coagulation screen
- Chest X-ray
- CT or ?US

- ERCP
- Fine needle aspiration biopsy after checking and correcting coagulation abnormalities

---

5. What do you think the patient is experiencing at this stage? How will you explain what you are thinking, and how your investigation protocol will sort out the different possibilities?

Phase 2

LFTs show raised SAP (850 IU/l), normal bilirubin, γGT and trans-aminases. Albumin 32 g/l. EUC all normal. Hb 88 g/l, normal wbc, platelets, coagulation parameters. CEA 5.6 u/l (normal <3.2), AFP normal. Iron studies normal. CT 6 × 4 cm mass replacing gall bladder; old calcified stone in gall bladder; multiple 1–3 cm filling defects right and left liver. ERCP some extrinsic compression of bile duct. Tumour fungating into duodenum laterally — biopsy reveals adenocarcinoma probably of gastrointestinal origin. FNA therefore not done.

1. What do you now consider the diagnosis to be? (Ca gall bladder)
2. How will you explain this to the patient and his wife?
3. Why is the patient anaemic? (anaemia of malignancy, duodenal invasion)
4. What treatment options will you discuss? (palliative care, chemotherapy, radiotherapy)
5. What answer will you give when they ask whether the condition can be cured?
6. What answers will you give to the questions 'Will any treatment do any good?' and 'What would you yourself have done?'
7. How will you deal with the following?

   a. A demand for another opinion.
   b. An insistence that the patient should travel to the Mayo Clinic for treatment.
   c. An admission by the patient that he is also being treated by a herbalist and that he proposes to visit a faith healer in the Philippines.
   d. A request for help with euthanasia when the suffering becomes too great.

Prognosis

From (a) your knowledge of the way that cancer behaves, and (b) your knowledge of the anatomy of the region, work out what symptoms the patient is likely to develop over the next few months. Then work out how you will answer the following questions from the patient and his wife.

1. How long have I got to live? (6–12 months)
2. What can I expect to suffer? (pain, anorexia, vomiting, GI bleeding, jaundice, cholangitis, anaemia, increasing fatigue)
3. What can be done to relieve these symptoms? (drugs, coeliac block, stenting, surgical bypass, transfusion, appetite stimulators)
4. How will I die? (increasing weakness, fatigue, pneumonia, blood loss)
5. Can I die at home?
6. What practical help can we get at home later in the illness?

Checklist

By the end of this episode, students should have learned or revised the following:

1. the biological and pathological features of adenocarcinoma of gastrointestinal origin;
2. the anatomy of the right upper quadrant of the abdomen, and the ways that it may be disrupted by 1;
3. an investigation protocol for a right upper quadrant mass.
4. some principles that may help in breaking bad news to patients;
5. some principles of palliative care for upper GI cancer;
6. some of the support services available for the terminally ill;
7. some insight into the nature of the experience of terminal illness.

Place in the curriculum

1 Years 3 and 4 in a four-year curriculum.

2. Built on formal teaching sessions in Years 1 and 2, including:
   a. anatomy of the abdomen;
   b. physiology of liver, gall bladder, biliary tree, pancreas, and gut;
   c. the nature and behaviour of cancer;
   d. the theory and practice of communication with patients, particularly the communication of bad news and probabilities;
   e. principles of palliative care.

Index